Interpersonal Trauma and its Consequences in Adulthood

Interpersonal Trauma and its Consequences in Adulthood

Edited by

Agnieszka Widera-Wysoczańska
and Alicja Kuczyńska

CAMBRIDGE
SCHOLARS

PUBLISHING

Interpersonal Trauma and its Consequences in Adulthood,
Edited by Agnieszka Widera-Wysoczańska and Alicja Kuczyńska

This book first published 2010

Cambridge Scholars Publishing

12 Back Chapman Street, Newcastle upon Tyne, NE6 2XX, UK

British Library Cataloguing in Publication Data
A catalogue record for this book is available from the British Library

ISBN (10): 1-4438-2400-3, ISBN (13): 978-1-4438-2400-2

TABLE OF CONTENTS

Part III: The Development of Personality Disorders

Part IV: Neurobiological Disorders

Part V: Psychological Trauma Treatment

List of Illustrations

LIST OF TABLES

INTRODUCTION

ALICJA KUCZYŃSKA AND AGNIESZKA WIDERA-WYSOCZAŃSKA

In this book we present studies on the influence of various forms of abuse experienced in childhood on the personal functioning of that individual in adulthood, including resulting life problems and personality and neurobiological disorders.

The source of this interpersonal psychological trauma is a traumatic event that is repetitive, chronic and complex in nature, and is caused by the action of a closely related person. Along with these traumatic events are included various types of neglect and violence, which a person may be subjected to from early childhood - in those times which are developmentally important for her/him - and then through the juvenile years, often up to the current moment of her/his life. Complex interpersonal psychological trauma occurs most frequently in a dysfunctional and pathological family. This causes the appearance of various types of symptoms, which can be very broadly divided, on one hand, into short and long term and, on the other, specific and unspecific. These symptoms, with their causes and consequences, can be either internal or external depending upon the extent to which they can be seen on the outside. The nature of these symptoms varies over one's entire life-span. They can accumulate, leading to secondary problems in life. When a person experiences extremely dramatic trauma they can lead to various personality disorders (e.g. borderline personality disorders, dissociation and psychopathic personality disorders) and to Complex Posttraumatic Stress Disorders (CPTSD). Interpersonal characteristics - chronic and complex traumatic events - go far beyond stressful events described in the classic PTSD (Criterion A). Traumatization of this type is extreme, often being life-threatening, emotionally horrifying, and physically and sexually violating. Symptoms of CPTSD also go beyond the triad of symptoms (intrusive reexperiencing, Criterion B; avoidance, Criterion C; and hyperarousal, Criterion D) described in PTSD. These include core problems such as affect dysregulation, structural dissociation, somatic dysregulation, an impaired self-concept and self-development, and disorganized attachment patterns as well as many other symptoms which are still the subject of scientific research and discussions.

We also describe psychotherapeutic issues connected with interpersonal trauma in our book. The issues contained in this part concern the sexologist experiences from work with perpetrators of sexual violence, problems connected with treatment of alcohol addicted people, partners remaining in conflicted relationship as well as parents who harm their children.

Since most of the presented studies are primarily concerned with the Polish population, the book may be an interesting example of the discussed issues as seen from the perspective of a society subject to a complex system and its mental transformations.

The book consists of five parts.

Part 1. The paper by Alicja Kuczyńska is a short introduction to interpersonal trauma issues. Analyzing the individual and social aspect of trauma, the author brings readers closer to understanding this phenomenon, gives some examples of factors that cause these kinds of experiences, and indicates sequels to them. The analysis will serve also to describe the general potential for trauma prevention and to help traumatized people, with particular consideration aimed at the psychologist's role.

Agnieszka Widera-Wysoczańska describes the main features and consequences of complex and chronic trauma and compares these features with simple trauma. She presents some examples of this kind of disorder from her practice. The author takes also a subject of intergenerational transmission of violence.

Part 2, "Dysfunctional relationships in adulthood" is devoted to events which affect the quality of relationships in adulthood. These events, which amount to chronic complex trauma, take place within the family and community in early childhood, adolescence, and adulthood. The article by Jowita Wycisk presents theoretical discussions about interpersonal traumatic events in their past and in their current life which cause young girls to become mothers too early.

The article by Irena Pospiszyl, based on empirical studies, describes past behaviors of women who are currently being beaten by their partners. It concerns extra-familial ways of functioning from childhood and adolescence - interests, social activities, and number of friends. The results confirm literature data which indicate that women who are beaten in relationships were socially passive in the past, although being professionally active in adult life. The article by A. Widera-Wysoczańska presents results of a qualitative study on the influence of the attachment of overprotective and non-protective mothers with their children on those children's partner selection in adulthood. This is placed in the context of emotional, physical, and sexual childhood abuse and over protectiveness.

Part 3, "The development of personality disorders", is devoted to the causes of the origin of borderline interpersonal disorders (BDP) and of their psychopathic structures.

The theoretical article by Lidia. Cierpiałkowska presents the causes of BDP, seen in traumatic relationships during childhood. The time of their appearance is considered.

The empirical article by Marylin. Korzekwa examines the causes of the appearance of dissociation in BPD and finds it in childhood abuse, parental addictions, the child's own addictions, disturbed relationships, and neurological problems with their their neurobiology, etiology and treatment.

The article by Beata Pastwa-Wojciechowska describes what kinds of childhood traumatic experiences occur in the lives of women and men with psychopathic personality structures which condemn them to domestic abuse. The influence of disturbed ties with the mother on the development of this disorder is highlighted.

Part 4, "Neurobiological disorders", deals with the influence of interpersonal trauma on a person's neurobiological functioning. The article by R. Gregurek presents research on the influence of war trauma (the war in Croatia) on brain functions in persons with PTSD. That by Olga Sakson-Obada demonstrates the influence of domestic abuse on physical numbness and sensitivity.

Part 5, "Psychological trauma treatment" focuses on practical questions about people who experienced interpersonal trauma. Most of the articles were devoted to trauma survivors. In the article by Alicja Kuczyńska and Alicja Strzelecka-Lemiech examine situational determinants of readiness for intervention by social workers and people who are not professionally involved in helping with domestic violence. The article by Agnieszka Widera-Wysoczańska presents the multiaspect principles concerning the philosophy and its methods of dealing with persons who experienced childhood interpersonal trauma and are suffering its consequences in adulthood. Dorota Dyjakon in her article presents the psychotherapy of alcoholics-perpetrators of domestic violence as a proposal which enriches the therapeutic offer for addicted people. It also gives attention to the special nature of problems which arise in an alcoholic family in relation to using violence by addicted people not only in an active phase of the disease but also after starting treatment. Finally, in the article by Maria Beisert we turn our attention to what kind of victimization persons who assist perpetrators of sexual abuse might be subjected to.

We thank Cambridge Scholars Publishing very much for the proposal to prepare a book devoted to interpersonal trauma and confidence shown to us in this manner. We were very honored and pleased for his opportunity to present the Polish thought to a wider reader on the issue. We give special thanks to the representative of the Cambridge Scholars Publishing, Carol Koulikourdi, for very kind cooperation and patience shown during the process of its preparation.

We invited many prominent authors to co-operate with us in the creation of the book.

There were three reviewers - prof. Grazyna Dolińska-Zygmunt, prof. Barbara Pilecka and prof. Kinga Lachowicz-Tabaczek - whose suggestions and comments have contributed greatly to the book. All these people we thank very much for such successful cooperation and commitment.

PART I

WHAT IS TRAUMA?

CHAPTER ONE

INDIVIDUAL AND SOCIAL ASPECTS OF TRAUMA

ALICJA KUCZYŃSKA

The paper is a short introduction to interpersonal trauma issues. Analyzing the individual, social and cultural aspect of trauma, the author brings readers closer to understanding this phenomenon, gives some examples of factors that cause these kinds of experiences, and indicates sequels to them. The analysis will serve also to describe the general potential for trauma prevention and for helping traumatized people, with particular consideration aimed at the psychologist's role.

The aim of this presentation is to introduce the problem of trauma. I would like to describe in short the types of traumatic events, the likelihood of experiencing them and reactions to them, as well as the general potential for helping people who have experienced trauma. I found it would be convenient to look at the issues both from the perspective of the individual as well as from the social aspects of trauma.

The notion of trauma stems from the Greek word *trauma* meaning a wound, and is colloquially regarded as referring to a psychological (traumatic) or bodily injury. Although the term appeared in published papers on psychology and medicine as early as the nineteenth century, systematic work aiming at establishing its definition and a more detailed role that experiences of this nature may play in the development of mental problems or disturbances was undertaken as late as the 1970's. The work concentrated on listing events that could potentially trigger adverse outcomes for the participants, characterizing these events and describing their psychological consequences. The result was the addition of a new category of mental disorders, - *Posttraumatic Stress Disorder* or PTSD - into the 1980 edition of the diagnostic classification system DSM-III. The major defining criteria was the notion of trauma understood as an unusually intensive and unwanted experience that involves actual or felt danger to one's life or health, evoked by direct contact of the individual with extreme, atypical life events (APA, 1980, p. 236). The experience results in a persistent re-experiencing of the traumatic event, avoidance of situations/stimuli associated with the trauma and persistent symptoms of increased arousal and anxiety. The official distinction of this new category of disturbances laid a good foundation for reviving the discussion on the essence and meaning of trauma, and undertaking intensive empirical attempts to explore this phenomenon. The results gathered from these studies brought two important findings. First, they proved that trauma is not such an infrequent phenomenon as had been previously assumed (Kessler et al., 1995; Breslau et al.,1998)[1], which resulted in a revised definition of trauma in the recent edition of classification DSM-IV-TR. The DSM-IV-TR refers to trauma as: 1) an experience of an event that involves actual or threatened death, serious injury to oneself or others, and 2) a response involving intense fear, helplessness, or horror (Oltmanns, Emery, 2007, p. 217). The findings also pointed to a wide range of traumatic events, including not only warfare, natural disasters, accidents or dramatic chance incidents, but also violence inflicted by others, rejection or betrayal, which in turn lead to an intensified revival of the trend of research on the kind of trauma that comes from another person, which is most frequently described as relational or interpersonal trauma.

The types of potentially traumatizing events

The number of events that are a potential source of human misfortunes is actually unlimited. They include not only natural disasters (flood, hurricanes, earthquakes), events caused by humans (plane or rail crashes, ship sinking or serious traffic accidents), acts of terror and warfare (such as participation in battle, imprisonment or being taken as a hostage, and torturing), but also interpersonal traumas. Although the term suggests that it encompasses all traumatic events (the source of which is another human being (including the death of a close person or threat to his or her life)[2] most researchers restrict the range of events under the heading of interpersonal trauma to ones where the perpetrator is another close person. They also pinpoint the intentions of the perpetrator, whose motivation is either the desire to hurt the other and/or the desire to pursue his or her own goals, irrespective of harm and costs to other people. Examples of this kind of phenomenon may be assault, battery, mutilation, rape or sexual abuse.

Although the subject of this monograph is interpersonal trauma, I would like to draw your attention to the fact that an attempt to describe the intentions of people participating in other traumatic events could have significance for better understanding the reactions of trauma victims and determining responsibility shared by the perpetrators of the events. For example, active participation in warfare or practicing harmful customs or rituals does not necessarily have to be originally related to the desire of hurting others. Usually such activities are associated with the intention of pursuing the goals of a group or with sustaining ways of functioning arising from the desire or necessity to belong to the group, and secure oneself appropriate, advantageous or at least fundamental living conditions within the group. Nevertheless, the intention is fulfilled irrespective of the harm and cost to other people.

The likelihood of experiencing trauma

At first it would seem that traumatic events are accidental by nature. However, the frequency of experiencing trauma by various people is not by chance and depends on many individual, social and cultural variables. It is more likely for people with a history of behaviour disorder, and for those who are anxious or poorly educated, but it is also likely for those coming from families where mental disorders occurred in the past or are present. Groups that are particularly at risk of traumatic events include people from social minorities and persons living in dangerous environments or areas of civil conflicts. Also, sex is found to be an important differential variable. The degree of exposure of women and girls, men and boys to a potential traumatic event depends on the type of event. A review by Tolin and Foa (2006) of 290 publications devoted to this problem proved that men and boys, more so than women and girls, frequently report experiences involving assaults, accidents, warfare, disasters and fire, serious illness, non-specific injuries or witnessing death and the wounding of others. On the other hand, women and girls more often than men experience assaults, sexual violence and abuse in childhood. Here, a question obviously arises as to what extent biological sex actually differentiates the likelihood of exposure to traumatic events, and what the role is of factors or mechanisms pertaining to biological sex, but accounting for its circumstances that are of a social and cultural nature.

Reactions to potential traumatic events and their consequences

Not everyone reacts to extreme events with such intense sensations as the trauma definition assumes. However, experiencing trauma involves the risk of acute stress disorder (ASD), posttraumatic stress disorder (PTSD) or complex posttraumatic stress disorder (CPTSD).

Diagnostic criteria of acute stress are in essence very similar to the above-described symptoms typical of PTSD, with the difference being that they also include dissociative symptoms (such as emotional numbness, derealisation, depersonalisation or dissociative amnesia) and should not persist longer than four weeks.

CPTSD is actually a new diagnostic unit proposed as a result of the study of people who survived multiple trauma of a cumulative nature. The prototype of the diagnostic criteria for this category of disorders stems from research on the consequences of a prolonged, recurrent trauma originating in childhood. The consequences of this kind of trauma influence the following aspects of functioning:

a) affect regulation (including difficulties in the regulation of anger as well as self-destruction)
b) alterations in attention and consciousness (dissociative symptoms)
c) alterations in self-perception (self-blame, guilt)
d) alterations in perception of the perpetrator (acceptance of the perpetrator's belief system)
e) alterations in relations with others (inability to trust others and lack of comfort/intimacy in relationships)
f) somatisation and/or medical conditions
g) alterations in the systems of meaning (sense of helplessness resulting from the impossibility of being understood by anyone) (Herman,1992a, 1992b, in: Courtois (2008).

Although it is assumed that no one is able to develop symptoms characteristic of ASD or PTSD without having experienced considerably intensive trauma, the experience of trauma itself is not a sufficient condition of PTSD. There have been attempts to predict depersonalization and emotional numbness (Bryant et al., 2000), on the basis of ASD symptoms, especially the ones that relate to re-experiencing the traumatic event. However, it is usually assumed that PTSD results from a combination of many factors, including pre-traumatic biological and personality features, the severity of the experienced harm, the manner in which emotional processing of the experience takes place, or the fact of having or not having received appropriate social support (Oltmanns, Emery, 2007). A meta-analysis of 68 publications by Ozer and her colleagues (2003) showed seven important predictors of the risk of PTSD. Most of the analysed factors are of an individual character, but the authors also considered one indirect factor and one social factor. These analysed factors are: experiencing at least one traumatic event, psychological adaptation before the examined trauma (including mental problems or disorder, such as depression or anxiety disorders), perception of life endangerment while experiencing trauma, a high level of emotional arousal during the stressful event and immediately afterwards, dissociative experiences, perceived social support after the experienced trauma, and the occurrence of mental illness in the family history.

Referring again to the results of the analysis by Tolin and Foa (2006), it could be added that, although they are less likely to be exposed to a potentially stressful event, the reactions of women are more intense, and as a result they more frequently develop symptoms of PTSD than do men.

Helping trauma survivors

Exposure to a potentially traumatic event does not always have to result in mental disorders. Many researchers believe that mental disorders may be prevented through appropriate resilience training and immediate crisis intervention. Obviously, the specificity of interpersonal trauma makes employment of the first form of prevention impossible. Hence crisis intervention is used, and in general it consists in describing or reenacting the painful experience for the victim of a traumatic event, and providing him or her with professional support. Although most studies show that immediate help reduces the risk of disorders occurring, the efficiency of one-time interventions has been challenged (Oltmanns, Emery, 2007). There is no evidence that escaping ASD or PTSD is truly the result of the intervention itself or is due to personality traits of the person subject to the potentially traumatic event - such as high self-esteem (Bryant et al., 2007; Stinson et al., 2008), self-efficacy (Leszczyńska et al., 2009), one's ability to cope in stressful situations or ego resiliency (Bonanno, 2008; conf. Staub et al., 2008).

The principal aim of therapy of ASD and PTSD patients is restoring them to the level of functioning in the period preceding the traumatic event. Peterson, Prout and Schwarz (1991: in Lis-Turlejska, 2002, p.102) distinguished four strategies common to all therapeutic proceedings. They include:

1. supporting adaptive abilities of coping
2. „normalization" of what the person perceives as disturbed
3. reduction of avoidance
4. changing the alteration of/changing the attribution of the meaning of trauma

Due to the specificity of CPTSD, the goal of therapy is bringing the person to the best possible way of functioning that may potentially be achieved in the face of prolonged and serious symptoms of sickness. The course of therapy is sequential, and consists in three stages (Courtois, 2008 p. 5-6):

1. The first step is devoted to the building of therapeutic alliance, working on affect regulation, education, providing security and achieving the ability to cope.
2. The achievement of the above-goals makes it possible to move to the second stage - that is, to the analysis and processing of the traumatic material, enabling the person to function in a less disturbed way.
3. The third step aims toward the consolidation and restructuring of life, allowing personal and social development to be reinforced by everyday life events.

Conducting therapy with trauma survivors involves many difficulties. They pertain both to the person who is the therapist, and the one who is in therapy. The major factor making therapy difficult on the part of the patient is the nature of his or her experience, especially when it concerns trauma experienced in the family (Herman, 1998; Briere, 1986, 1998; Suchańska, 1998; Courtois, 2008). The symptoms of the principal disorders themselves may hinder communication and excessively increase vigilance or sensitivity to the therapist's behavior. There are also frequent co-occurrences of somatic conditions (vascular circulation, gastroenterological problems, diabetes, and oncological diseases) and mental illness (depression, substance abuse disorders, antisocial symptoms, and borderline personality disorders) (conf. Lis-Turlejska, 2002; Oltmanns, Emery, 2007; Elhai et al., 2007; Kendall-Tackett, 2009).

The basic factor hindering therapy on the part of the therapist is the necessity of being very competent, as lack of competence brings about the risk of re-victimisation of the client. Such a lack is brought about by still quite limited possibilities of attaining necessary therapeutic skills. Therefore, the major challenge that the psychologists are confronted with is acquiring knowledge on trauma, on the experiences of people who have suffered it, and on the possibilities of helping them, as well as spreading information and generously sharing it with everyone who is willing to receive it (conf. Miller, 2007; Kazdin, 2009).

In presenting the individual and social aspects of trauma, I wished to show that the science of trauma is first of all a science regarding humans. While it is humans who experience traumatic events (and often directly or indirectly are also the perpetrators of them), it is also only humans who can help others in overcoming the consequences of dramatic experiences and act towards creating a better world. The words of a Romanian philosopher, Emile Cioran (2004, p.126) may guide us in doing so:

> „I am reflected in your eyes, and so are you in mine. Each of us is reflected in the eyes of the other. The whole world is looking at itself in the tears of each of us. As in the faces of old icons, we remain devoutly bent over our cloudy clearness - radiating, but not transparent.
>
> Let the tears become our true mirror. There our suffering and ecstasies will unite. Is there anything better than a shed tear for being the mirror of the one who has lost his paradise?
>
> It is in tears only that we regain our face.
>
> And since the tears flow out from the depth of the human being, they are like a calling from another paradise, the one we will enter after our final moment, after our second tear".

Notes

[1] Research findings suggest that trauma is experienced by people living in various countries (e.g. Japan [Allard, 2009], Mexico [Norris et al., 2003[, Sweden [Frans et al., 2005] or Poland [Statystyka Sądowa i Penitencjarna Ministerstwa Sprawiedliwości, 1998]), irrespective of age (Herzberger, 2002; Badura-Madej et al.,2000; Dobrzyńska-Mesterhazy, 1996; Czapczyńska, 2007; Courois, 2009).
[2] The review by Cabizuc and colleagues (2009) of sixteen papers showed that there is an increased risk of PTSD among parents of children who are chronically ill or subject to intensive medical procedures. Since one of the consequences of PTSD may also be a restriction of parental competence in the caretaking role during this difficult period for the parents and their children, the authors postulate the necessity of early diagnosis of parental functioning in order to prevent extremely important negative outcomes.

CHAPTER TWO

INTERPERSONAL TRAUMA AS CHRONIC AND COMPLEX

AGNIESZKA WIDERA-WYSOCZAŃSKA

Interpersonal trauma belongs to complex and chronic injuries, and it arises in connection with experiencing different types of abuse. In this article I wish to show the characteristics of chronic and complex trauma and compare them with those of a simple trauma. I describe the types of families which provide environments for interpersonal trauma and the types of abuse which contribute to complex interpersonal suffering. The perpetrator, usually close to the person wronged, is responsible for the abuse. Specific consequences (that a person suffered a specific type of abuse) and non-specific symptoms (that a person suffered some abuse) resulting from trauma depends on the age at which a person experiences it. These sufferers change over time (*life-span*); their traumas lead to secondary problems of life, while the accumulation of complex interpersonal traumas can lead to various disorders, including complex Post-Traumatic Stress Disorder (CPTSD). These consequences become an intermediary in the transmission of violence from generation to generation, and require specific therapy.

Psychological traumatic stressor events

To more clearly understand the concept of "trauma" a distinction was made between the traumatic event and the person's subjective reaction to it. The reaction is made during one's lifetime or in the immediate aftermath of the experience (peritraumatic) or as post-traumatic (occurring weeks, months, years afterwards) (Weathers, Keane, 2007). In trauma specialists opinion, the word "psychological trauma" applies only to events that are stressful and negative for the person. Responding to this event is defined as post-traumatic consequence occurring in the form of reactions, problems and disorders. Let me begin with a description of psychological characteristics of types of traumatic events.

1. Simple traumatic events

The definition of a traumatic event, presented in PTSD A criterion contained in DSM-IV-TR (APA, 2000), shows a traumatic event as one which threatens health, life or the physical integrity of the person directly involved or of someone who is closely related. A person can experience the event, be a witness of it or hear about it. He/she can bear the consequences of the event or be a witness of its consequences, but not be threatened (Criterion A1). In addition, the reaction of the person is accompanied by anxiety, helplessness and horror (Criterion A2). Potentially traumatic events include natural disasters, including earthquakes, hurricanes, floods, or man-made disasters, such as car or aircraft accidents, a ship sinking, an explosion, and wars and diseases as well as physical or sexual assault by stranger, robbery, kidnapping , or being held hostage (Briere, Spinazzola, 2005; Briere, Scott, 2006; Van Hooff, Mc Farlane, Baur, Abraham, Barnes, 2009).

Table 2-1. Simple traumatic event according to PTSD, Criterion A "exposure to trauma" (DSM-IV-TR: APA, 2000).

The criterion of "A" with PTSD	Examples
A 1.1. A person who has witnessed or experienced events in which death or a threat of death occurred, where there is a threat to physical health or serious injury to a person.	Natural disasters: - earthquakes - floods - volcanoes The catastrophe caused by a human being: - Transport accidents with multiple victims: aviation, railway, ship, bus - Transport accidents with one or more victims: auto-mobile, motorcycle - Fires of houses or other buildings - Collapse of buildings Military actions: - War - Torture Interpersonal abuse (occasional) made by foreigners: - Rapes - Physical attack

	- Beatings Attack by an animal: - e.g. a dog
A 1.2. A person was a witness of the consequences of catastrophic events, but he/she was never threatened.	- Seeing bodies of people who died in a transport accident or during natural disasters - Watching a man being beaten - Exposure of emergency staff to the trauma
A 1.3. A person confronted with the consequences of a threat to the life of a close relative.	- Information that somebody we love or someone who is important to us was seriously injured or died in unknown circumstances, it is not known what happened to his/her body - Kidnapping, loss of the beloved one, and lack of knowledge of his/her fate

According to the response to severe stress (F43) described in ICD-10 (International Classification of Diseases) (2000) a traumatic event is described as a stressful event or situation, either short or long, of an exceptionally threatening or catastrophic nature which produces a severely negative experience for almost everybody (Tab.2-2).

Table 2-2. Simple traumatic events according to ICD-10 (2000).

In order to recognise the "reaction to severe stress" disorder category, it is necessary to experience one of the following causal factors:
1. extremely stressful life event, physical or psychological, caused by a severe reaction to stress 2. significant life change leading to permanent and painful situations that causes adaptation disorders 3. genesis and severity of acute stress depend mainly on onto-genetic sensitivity and one's ability to cope with stress 4. stressor causing disorder, which disorganises the social reference frame of an individual (bereavement, separation), or interferes with wider social support systems and values (migration, refugee status) 5. stressor can be associated with a significant stage of development for an individual or with a crisis of development (parenting, retirement, etc.).

The same event need not be traumatic for everyone. The objective description of a traumatic event presented in the A criterion should be supplemented by a subjective interpretation of the event made by the person. The element of this subjective interpretation refers to the inclusion of an emotional reaction in the form of fear, helplessness and horror in the A criterion of PTSD (DSM-IV–TR: APA, 2000). It was therefore concluded that reaction to traumatic stress can come from real emotional or physical abuse, and from external threats due to the subjective interpretation of those events.

The description by Lenore Terr (1991, 1994) of two types of traumatic events was a landmark step in defining traumatic events, ranging from a one-off situation to recurring events. Type I includes a single-incident trauma, which is sudden and unexpected. By contrast, type II is a complex or repetitive trauma for a chronic, recurrent, and accumulating experience, which can be anticipated and expected by the person. This type of traumatic event was described by Terr (1988) to show the specificity of interpersonal trauma experienced by a person in his/her childhood in the family.

According to ICD-10 (ICD-10, 2000), type II trauma is described as less severe psychosocial stresses called "life events" which can contribute to a number of abnormalities found in various categories of ICD-10 (particularly for adjustment disorders, F43.2). The very occurrence of a life event is not sufficient to explain the emergence of the disorder, as formation of its clinical picture also depends on the patient's own sensitivity.

The foundations for more precise defining interpersonal, complex and chronic, traumatic events were established in the following manner.

2. Interpersonal, complex and chronic traumatic events

Psychological interpersonal trauma incurs in connection with experiencing different types of abuse and negligence, and most often occurs in a dysfunctional and pathological family. This event is *interpersonal* and is connected with a specific type of bond, mainly a dysfunctional one (ambivalent, avoidant, disorganised, dissociative: Bowlby, 1973). It is the result of people who are close and important to the person wronged; moreover, the abuse being traumatic event is done deliberately and intentionally. Such an active (direct) perpetrator hurts the person manipulating him/ her, seducing, addicting emotionally, and subjecting the sufferer in order to use - secretly and with impunity - other abuse (e.g. emotional, physical, and sexual). Causing harm to the person, the perpetrator evokes a feeling of betrayal and undermines trust in primary relationships. The passive offender, the second parent, care-giver or person on whom the child depends, and does not offer protection and support. This situation causes a second injury: loss of basic confidence and a feeling of betrayal from the care-giver (betrayal trauma). The closer the relationship between perpetrator and the person wronged, the more serious its consequences can be.

The *complexity* of traumatic events indicates that during the same period of life a person experiences both various types of abuse and negligence. Their *chronic* nature means that traumatic events such as emotional, physical or sexual abuse, contravening intimate barriers and chemical dependency are repeated several times, both in the same time frame as well as for many subsequent years. A person could be subjected to these stressful events from early childhood, during those periods which are developmentally important, then throughout his/her youth - and often to the current moment. It affects the victim's *development* in important moments (Ford, Courtois, 2009). The traumatic event as a result becomes an "*everyday", ordinary human experience*: in childhood and/or adulthood.

The trauma is *foreseeable*, a person knows that offender will be abusive again; but it is also *unpredictable*, because they do not know exactly when, where, how and to what extent. The person lives in an atmosphere of constant tension and fear. The inability to predict and control the hazard leads to generalised anxiety, a generalised sense of insecurity within the whole environment. It is related to a compulsive need by the child, as well as by other family members, to recognize signals of impending abuse. Complex trauma tends to *increase* and *expand*. When one type of traumatic event occurs in a family, for example emotional abuse, it is likely to lead to its intensification and, consequently, to the occurrence of other, even more drastic, types of abuse, including, for instance, beatings or sexual abuse. Leading to the threats to the life of individual family members (severity of offender behaviours and suicidal risk tendencies increase) can be the next step (Walker, 2009).

A complex trauma is *direct* when a child or other person is hurt and *indirect* when the child observes - being a witness - other people in the family being hurt. Another trauma feature refers to a lowered degree of *reflectivity* of passive and active perpetrators. The lower the reflectivity of people responsible for abuse towards a child and other family members, the less chance to improve the situation in a family, and therefore to stop abuse.

Interpersonal, chronic, and complex traumatic events appears short or long term specific and non-specific *consequences* in the lives of people, the dynamic nature of which changes over a life time (*life - span*), if it accumulates it can lead to secondary life problems. Persons subject to extremely drastic trauma can lead to various personality disorders, especially complex post-traumatic stress disorders (Tab.2-3).

Table 2-3. Features of complex and chronic interpersonal traumatic events (Wysoczańska - Widera, 2007).

Features	Description
Interpersonal character and bonds	traumatic events are actions of people who are close and important to the person wronged, abuse is done deliberately and intentionally
Complexity	the person experiences various types of abuse and negligence at the same time
Chronic character	traumatic events are repeated several times: (a) in one period and (b) for many years of a person's life.
Commonness and everyday character	the abuse becomes a normal life event
Developmental nature	it affects the development of a person, the person is subjected to stressful events from early childhood, in developmentally important periods of time
Predictability Unpredictability	certainty that harm will be done again uncertainty as to the place, time and method
Loss of control	no control over the behaviour of a perpetrator, oneself, and the environment in which the person will be found
Progression	severity of a particular type of abuse and, in turn, of other forms of abuse, becoming more and more drastic until life-threatening occur
Directness and indirectness	a child or other person is hurt or, as a witness, observes people close to him/her being hurt
Reduced level of reflexivity	the smaller reflectivity of passive and active perpetrators, the less chance to change the situation in the family and the greater the severity of abuse
Dynamism of effects in the course of a person's life	severity and nature of the consequences dynamically change over a lifetime (life-span), can accumulate and lead to secondary life problems for people undergoing drastic trauma, can lead to various personality disorders especially to complex post-traumatic stress disorders

Terr (1994) and Finkelhor (1986) consider that our whole life can be shaped by early trauma, whether or not it is remembered by the person. Early interpersonal trauma causes more complex psychopathology than later interpersonal traumatisation. The closer in proximity a person is to the perpetrator, the more serious the consequences are upon that person's life. Interpersonal trauma causes more problems than trauma not caused by another person. Difficulties in expressing emotion and showing trust often become a source of problems in adult life; as a consequence, it may affect the building of close and lasting relationships in, bringing up children.

Comparison of complex chronic trauma with simple trauma

As made clear from the above-description, the characteristics of interpersonal, chronic and complex trauma goes beyond the distressing events described in a classic PTSD (A criterion, DSM-IV-TR: APA, 2000) occurrence. The difference between type I and type II traumas presented in Table 2-4 results from the difference of stress events experienced by a person, and it affects the type of symptoms appearing in that person.

Table 2-4. Comparison of type I and type II traumatic events.

Complex chronic trauma (type II)	Simple acute trauma (type I)
Complex - several types of abuse at one time	One event
Chronic - lasts for a long time	"Dose" - lasts for a limited time, often a one-off Exposure to recurring natural disasters (such as the earthquakes)
As a result of its repeatability, it becomes a "normal", ordinary and everyday experience	It goes beyond everyday experience
Predictable and repetitive - all the time (the mere fact of occurrence) Unpredictable - time, place, form Predictability and volatility occur together Uncontrolled	Predictable and repeatable (e.g. earthquakes in a seismically active place) Unpredictable (e.g. transportation accidents, terrorism) Predictability and volatility occur together Uncontrolled
Interpersonal - all the time: the perpetrator is a close, trusted person from whom safety, love, intimacy, support is expected but intentionally- and deliberately-done wrong occurs	Interpersonal character - sometimes: 1. when the perpetrator is a stranger, from whom security is not expected and who conducts a single attack: (such as rape and a beating in the street, torture, or war) or

	2. when there is personal error - such as bad design of a house which collapses, bad construction of a dam which breaks, or lack of providing information about an upcoming natural disaster or terrorist attack Lack of interpersonal character - natural disaster (e.g. earthquake, tornado, hurricanes, floods, fire)
- Directness - life or health of a particular person is threatened, such the person himself/herself being beaten - Indirectness - he/she is a witness of events or their consequences (sees a close person being beaten up and sustaining injuries) - Interpersonal traumatic effect - bereavement and mourning, loss of home due to having to move out when the offender is allowed to stay in it, lack of social support, loss of close ties	- Directness - life or health of a person is threatened: car accident or flooding - Indirectness - he/she witnesses the event and its consequences, sees a close person whose health and life are endangered or are killed, and observes the consequences of the traumatic event. - Interpersonal traumatic effect - bereavement and mourning, loss of home, for example due to a fire
The beginning - most often childhood, but also adolescence or adulthood (abuse between partners)	It can occur at various ages in a person's life
Often we do not know the state "before" the trauma or the state "after " the trauma due to its chronic character and very early occurrence in the life of a person	The state "before" the trauma and "after" the trauma is known; it is a one-time event, although it can persist for some time, and sometimes it is repetitive in character (e.g. volcanic eruption)

We can distinguish between an objective event and its subjective understanding by the person. Every person reacts differently to stressful events in their life, and these reactions are considered as defence mechanisms and means of dealing with trauma.

The family as the environment of interpersonal trauma

There are three basic forms of the family: functional, dysfunctional and pathological. The functional family can be characterised by the fact that behaviours, roles, principles, values and beliefs existing within it meet basic and higher needs of all family members and enables their emotional, cognitive, social, behavioural, moral and spiritual development to the extent potentially possible for them. There are conflicts in the family but they are effectively addressed with conclusions drawn from them and brought to life. Family members are open to other people, flexible and reflective, willing to reach for help provided by relatives, friends and professionals. Reflective parents know that they are responsible for changes in the family. It seems that in these families there is little risk of recurring abuse in subsequent generations because it is stopped rather soon after it occurs.

Most families in which there is interpersonal, chronic and complex traumatic events (various forms of abuse) are dysfunctional. In these families - due to introduced and applied behaviours, roles, principles, values and beliefs - higher needs of family members are not sufficiently satisfied. Typically, their emotional, cognitive, social, behavioural, moral and spiritual development can remain below potential developmental capabilities of both children and parents.

Adult family members (care-givers) have problems in taking responsibility for the conditions of a family; therefore - to make a family function in some fashion - they pass on the task to their own children, who unconsciously adopt different roles imposed upon them to allow the family to survive. These care-givers have problems with their own reflectivity and flexibility, so family conflicts are not resolved in a timely manner or at all. Cumulative emotions can be seen in the form of growing, increasingly drastic, abuse. Children do not learn to cope with interpersonal conflicts; they lose control over themselves and the world as their sense of helplessness increases. If at the appropriate time, adults within a family did not respond to the abuse, and the behaviour associated with hurting others tends to increase, the family can become pathological.

It is characterised by a very wide intensity of various forms of abuse at the same time. The family does not meet basic and higher needs of its members. Moreover, their health and life in all the areas of operation listed above are seriously at risk because of parental addictions, abuse, and physical negligence or sexual abuse. Members of the family usually develop below their potential capabilities.

A great number of traumatic events which comprise interpersonal, complex chronic trauma and create a situation of abuse can occur in dysfunctional and pathological families (Type II trauma, Terr, 1991; Widera-Wysoczańska, 2007). There are three basic forms of abuse: emotional, physical and sexual, which set up foundations for numerous other traumas. These include, among other things, impaired relations with the parent, abuse and emotional negligence, abandonment, emotional and physical abuse, sexual abuse with intimate physical touching, sexual abuse without touching, emotional sexual abuse, overprotection which can be both emotional and sexual abuse, parental addiction to chemicals (alcohol, medicines, drugs), emotional and/or physical separation or divorce of the care-givers, wife or girlfriend stalking by the partner with emotional and physical or sexual abuse but as a result of domestic abuse, parent's experience of pathological grief after the loss of a loved one, and dysfunctional reactions of care-givers to the chronic illness of a child or other family member. There is also "fuzzy abuse", seen as unimportant as no one wants to take responsibility for it and which is difficult to diagnose (Table 2-5., Widera-Wysoczańska, 2010).

Table 2-5. Types of abuse as traumatic events in the family.

Types of abuse	Types of behaviour	
Disturbed attachment with mother and father		
Dissociative attachment		
Emotional	-abuse due to relationships of the offender with the victim	- direct and indirect
	-abuse in the kind of perpetrator's behaviour	- an adult towards a child - an adult towards another adult
	-parent's negligence towards a child	
Physical	-abuse in view of the kind of perpetrator's behaviour:	- passive - active
	-abuse in view of the person wronged:	- direct - indirect
	-parent's negligence towards a child	

Sexual abuse	-in a view of the origin of perpetrator -in view of the kind of perpetrator's behaviour towards a victim	- in-the-family (biological incest) - out-of-the-family, including (psychological incest) direct - with intimate touching and perpetration - sexual without touching - emotional and verbal sexual abuse indirect - procuration - acceptance of abuse against the child which the care-taker knows about - lack of response to abuse against the child which is not accepted by the care-taker - negligence of sex education
Over-protection	- intrusive control - sexual - Munchausen's by proxy	
Stalking	-emotional and physical aggressive behaviours of offender	-enters the house violently -destroying a car and property of the person persecuted -writing anonymous letters -making repeated phone calls -intimidating by threatening to commit suicide if a person does not do what the offender wants

addiction by parent (s) to:	- alcohol - medicines - drugs and other chemical agents - pornography
Separation or divorce of parents:	- emotive - physical
Abandonment - by euro-immigrant families	
Pathological grief experienced by a parent after the loss of a loved one	
Pathological reactions of care-takers to a chronic illness of a child or other family member	
Fuzzy abuse and others	

Life - span consequences of children and adults

When a child experiences domestic abuse, immediate reactions to stress occur. The symptoms which occur during and immediately after the abuse are regarded as healthy reactions as they variously protect an individual against currently experienced harm (Briere, 1992; Briere Scott, 2006; Courtois, 1998 and Ford, Courtois, 2009). But when these symptoms persist longer in one's emotional, cognitive, behavioural, social or somatic sphere or after several years appear in the form of life problems, they hamper a person's functioning because they are not adapted to new circumstances. Every person reacts individually, but a child's chronic and complex nature of the traumatic events does not give him/her time for recovery and integration. It is known that dysfunctional behaviours of these children spread outside their homes into the environment they live in, including relationships with peers in kindergarten or school or in the backyard. A beaten child can beat up others; sexually abused ones can release tension by duplicating these behaviours towards their peers. If they are not provided help, these reactions turn into long-term consequences until finally they enter adulthood with secondary problems that affect the conduct of these adult persons towards their partners and children.

The reaction to trauma can be best understood from the perspective of development, which focuses on changes in their adaptive and non-adaptive forms of dealing with traumatic events. This approach not only places symptoms in the lifespan of a particular person, but also takes into account the multi-generational process of transferring abuse and its symptoms (Widera-Wysoczańska, 2010).

The consequences of chronic trauma can be seen immediately after the injury and then for the whole life of a person. With some people there are only short-term consequences which quickly disappear without further recurrences. For others - after some time - they are not visible "outside", but as "inner" symptoms still influence the person's life. The short-term consequences can become long-term and can have chronic form: be delayed and onset after a few months (at least 6 months after the stressor, according PTSD, DSM-IV-TR: APA, 2000) or years after the traumatic situation, may be the symptoms with reemission which means that despite long periods of good health, symptoms can return in the situation when stress resembling the original traumatic events (Friedman, 2001). In the course of time symptoms could change into secondary life problems. Typically, a person with difficulty combine these problems with the original traumas. All the more so since these people have to react to relatively recent and current stressful situations and crises that stem from injuries suffered in various stages of person's life, from childhood to adulthood (Briere, 2004).

An adult who suffered abuse as a child needs significantly more time to recover and to minimize the cumulative consequences of repeated traumatic stresses. The more the person experiences traumatic events, the more post-traumatic symptomatology he/she will have.

Disorders as a consequence of abuse suffered in childhood

As a result of interpersonal, chronic trauma experienced in childhood, there can be a variety of symptoms and disorders occurring as well as numerous subjective feelings and meanings that are not easy to describe in a categories. Symptoms are treated as a pathology when they become a clinical manifestation of problems related to traumatic events and appear in the form of various post-traumatic disorders. Complex post-traumatic stress disorders (PTSD Complex, Herman, 1992a), also known as Disorders of Extreme Stress, not otherwise specified (DESNOS, Herman, Van der Kolk, 1987; Pelcovitz, Van der Kolk, Roth, Madel, Kaplan, Resich, 1997; Van der Hart, Nijenhuis, Steele, 2006; and Van der Kolk, Roth, Pelcovitz, Sunday, Spinazolla, 2005) can occur among others not mentioned in DSM-IV. CPTSD and DESNOS are created to specially describe adults (Ford, Courtois, 2009). CPTSD symptoms go beyond the symptoms (intrusive re-experiencing, avoidance and hyperarousal) described in "classic" PTSD. They include problems, such as: affect de-regulation, structural dissociation, somatic de-regulation, impaired self-concept and self development, and disorganised attachment patterns (Herman, 1992).

Acording Ford and Courtois (2009) the following can be included as "less specific" problems and personality disorders resulting from interpersonal trauma in one's childhood: traumatic stress personality disorder (TrSPD) or post-traumatic personality disorder (PPD), types: disorganised, similar to the abuse/attachment model of complex traumatic stress disorders (Brown, 2009) and organised, involves self-deregulation similar to DESNOS and social avoidance but without fundamental loss or fluctuations in trust and security (Ford, Courtois, 2009). Moreover, in the last several years developmental trauma disorder (DTD) affecting children is described as their subjective reaction to a traumatic event occurring during their development (Van der Kolk, 2005; Courtois, Ford, 2009). DTD is described in children by means of 1. deregulation which appears in one or two spheres (emotional, cognitive, somatic, social, behavioural, and attributive) and using 2. convictions resulting from abandonment, experiencing betrayal and abuse (Ford, Courtois, 2009).

For people with a history of interpersonal trauma - alongside CPTSD - at least one more psychiatric disorder is often diagnosed. Friedman (2001) point that in order to diagnose severe comorbid disorders, they must be independent of each other, and the diagnosis of one should not increase the likelihood of another (Ford, Courtois, 2009; Briere, 2006) .

The most frequently occurring symptoms and disorders coexisting with complex PTSD refer to dissociations occurring as mechanisms, habits and dissociative identity disorders described as DID in DSM-IV-TR (APA, 2000) and in ICD-10 (2000) as a dissociative disorder (Putnam, 1997). Dissociation is described in DSM-IV-TR (APA, 2000) as a disruption in usually integrated functions of consciousness, memory, identity or perception of the environment. As a consequence of interpersonal trauma somatoform responses and disorders as well conversion reaction can occur, which are physical or bodily symptoms that are strongly influenced by psychological factors, particularly those which have been linked to a history of childhood trauma. In ICD-10 (2000) they are described as neurotic disorders occurring in somatic form (F40), including anxiety disorders as various phobias (simple, social and agoraphobia) and anxiety disorders and somatic-like disorders (F45). The frequency of occurrence of fatigue, exhaustion, headaches or chest pain, and weakening of the immune system intensifies. The symptoms occurring in somatisation disorder described in DSM IV-TR (APA, 2000) refer to pain in the gastrointestinal, sexual, and neurological systems and they cannot be explained based on medical phenomena alone (Widera-Wysoczańska, 2006a). In contrast, only one physical complaint for which no medical explanation can be found can occur in undifferentiated somatoform disorder. Disorders of conversion (paralysis, loss of ability to speak, abnormal movements, deafness, blindness, seizures) refer to symptoms or deficits affecting voluntary motor or sensory functions that suggest a neurological or other general medical condition, but which cannot be fully explained medically (APA, 2000).

Mood disorders (affective) in the form of mild, moderate or severe depressive episodes (F32 in ICD-10, 2000) or recurrent depressive disorders (F33) or dysthymia (F34.1) and dysphoria are one of the most common forms of post-traumatic responses. In DSM-IV-TR (APA, 2000), mood disorders occur in the form of mood episodes, depressive disorders (in the form of single episodes and recurrent states) and dysthymia disorders. Complicated or traumatic grief can also occur (Briere, Scott, 2006). As trauma is often related to danger and vulnerability, post-traumatic outcomes often involve symptoms of anxiety. Such responses according DSM-IV-TR (2000) can be divided into three clusters: generalised anxiety, panic attacks, and post-traumatic phobias.

Women more often than men experience eating disorders (F50 according to ICD-10; 307.1 and 307.51 in DSM-IV-TR), including anorexia (anorexia nervosa) following emotional abuse, and bulimia (bulimia nervosa) as a result of frequent sexual abuse suffered in childhood. Especially after sexual abuse as well as other drastic forms of abuse, the following are typical: sexual dysfunctions (F52) according to ICD-10 and in DSM-IV-TR (APA, 2000) called sexual disorders, paraphilias and personality disorders (gender identity) in children or adolescents and adults, including gender identity disorders (F64, ICD-10, 2000) and sexual preferences (F65, ICD-10), or otherwise, unspecified (DSM-IV-TR: APA, 2000).

Other disorders include abnormal behaviours in the form of hyper-kinetic (motor hyperactivity complexes, F90, ICD-10), chemical addiction (alcohol, drugs, sleeping pills) and anti-social or dis-social disorders (F60.2, for ICD-10, 2000; 301.7 DSM -IV-TR, 2000).

There is a clear correlation between complex PTSD and borderline personality disorder and it occurs in 60-80% of women who experienced childhood sexual abuse and in patients after acute trauma (DSM-IV-TR, 2000; ICD-10, 2000; Herman, Perry & van der Kolk, 1989). DSM-IV describes borderline personality disorder as a chronic disturbance in which there is a pervasive instability pattern of interpersonal relationships, self-mage, and affects, and marked impulsiveness beginning in early adulthood and present in a variety of contexts (APA, 2000). A number of studies indicate that borderline personality disorder is generally associated with severe and extended childhood trauma, neglect, or loss (Herman, Perry, van der Kolk, 1989).

Social and family relationships deteriorate, irritability and nervousness increase, satisfaction with being together decreases, and marital problems and family arguments intensify. Unfortunately, due to the modular family the level of social support decreases, which is relevant in the process of recovery.

Intergeneration transmission

Interpersonal abuse and its consequences can be passed from generation to generation. Several factors can be distinguished which make up the self-propelling circle of abuse: social, family, personal and biological (Widera-Wysoczańska, 2010). Social values, beliefs, myths, and behaviour affect the conduct of caretakers in families towards each other and their children. When it comes to abuse, complex and chronic traumas experienced by family members launch processes of coping with abuse, which operate effectively at the time of its experiencing, but if the person continues in life to use these methods towards his/her own children and partner, they become destructive.

Long-term consequences maintain the cycle of abuse. In addition, trauma causes changes in the brain which are the basis of overly passive or aggressive behaviour expressed in the environment and that affect the degree to which these experiences are remembered.

Intermediate phenomena at the social level in the transmission of abuse refer to social learning, which is related to modeling more powerful and dominant. Abuse affects the learning of values, myths, beliefs and social conduct, while it accuses the victim and supports the offender. At the family level, intermediate factors refer to various forms of abuse. These factors refer to characteristics of parents and their mutual relationships, to psychological characteristics of the active offender (directly applying the abuse) and passive offender (not supporting and not protecting the wronged child), to relationships between the child's care-takers; they build a dysfunctional relationship with the child, with family rules, roles, and the child's expectations; they create a lack of skills for protecting children against abuse, even after its disclosure, and encourages denials of family abuse. At the personal level, they include denial defence mechanisms, and dissociation - in particular, de-realisation and depersonalisation, symptoms of PTSD such as avoidance, numbness, anger transferred from offenders to others (partner, their children, and foreigners), memory problems, and reduced empathy towards oneself and the person one hurts. In addition, there are the syndrome of helplessness, the stockholm syndrome, denials as defence mechanisms, and problems in building relationships with loved ones - one's children or partner including premature motherhood, or getting into a relationship with a violent man. At the biological level, brain changes occur in the hippocampus, thalamus, limbic system, cerebellum, frontal cortex, and insula. They are responsible for memory, agitation, or stupor when they are under the influence of threats, the inability to integrate traumatic memories with one's current life, or in blunted ways of feeling emotions.

Features of psychotherapy

The specificity of symptoms and problems arising from interpersonal traumas of experienced as chronic and complex, affect the type of interventions undertaken during therapy. To help a person, we diagnose symptoms that appear throughout the client's life, from childhood until therapy. We proceed while at the same time recognizing his/her current situation in the family and the environment. We look at the structure of the family of origin and at the current one - to the roles, rules, beliefs and above all risk factors related to the emergence and maintenance of various forms of domestic abuse. This form of therapy requires knowledge of how the human being has functioned from birth to death, and in various aspects of the person's life (The specificity of therapy will be discussed in part 5).

PART II

DYSFUNCTIONAL RELATIONSHIPS IN ADULTHOOD

CHAPTER THREE

TEENAGE MOTHERHOOD AND ITS CONNECTION WITH EXPERIENCING INTERPERSONAL ABUSE

JOWITA WYCISK

The aim of this article is to highlight the links between experiences of interpersonal abuse and premature motherhood. Using the term "premature", I mean motherhood of teenage girls. As in most cases the fact that a teenager becomes a mother is neither an act of her will, nor does it result from the fact of her being prepared for this role in any way. And, what is more, it is not the fruit of a steady and mature relationship; therefore it is regarded as a developmentally unpunctual event (Brzezińska 2003). It is also clear that these statements apply more to girls aged fourteen or fifteen rather than to eighteen or nineteen year-old women (to whom they may not apply at all) who terminate their education and decide to start up a family. However, because of the availability of empirical studies, where teenage mothers are usually generally treated as a homogenous group, this paper will be devoted to girls and women who are nineteen and younger when they become mothers

Teenage motherhood is certainly not a common phenomenon in Poland, and it is possible that for this reason it infrequently (and only recently) has attracted the attention of psychologists or researchers representing other fields of the humanities. Whenever it does occur, however, it usually addresses the way a young mother copes with the analyzed situation (in such cases teenage motherhood is considered as a difficult situation, conf. Więcławska, 2005), as well as with her psychological functioning during the pregnancy, delivery and puerperium (Bidzan, 2007), with the socio-pedagogical aspects of early motherhood (conf. Skowrońska, 2009), and its psychosocial consequences (Kościelska, 1998).

With respect to the diagnosis of the reasons for the occurrence of this phenomenon in Poland, attention is focused more frequently on the issues of insufficient sexual education (undoubtedly requiring many changes in our country[1]) and the early age of first sexual activity rather than on psychological or social factors. This has become an easy target for those who, even in their official statements as politicians[2], eagerly condemn girls who become sexually active early in their lives. However, many foreign studies show that an important factor increasing the risk of premature pregnancy is the abuse experienced earlier in life by girls and young women. Becoming familiar with the reported results should sensitize us (especially persons working with juvenile mothers) to the role of interpersonal violence and its consequence in the form of premature motherhood in Poland. However, before presenting the results of foreign studies and explaining the nature of the relationships between the discussed phenomena, I will present the data concerning the scale of teenage motherhood in Poland.

Teenage mothers - how big of a phenomenon are we talking about?

According to a report published in 2007 by the United Nations Development Programme and the Polish Ministry of Health, the number of teenage girls giving birth to children in Poland in the last sixteen years has been steadily declining (table 2-1). The frequency of deliveries among teenage girls is measured by the rate of fertility, namely the number of live births in one year in 1000 women aged fifteen to nineteen. In 2004 the rate of fertility was 14‰, which constitutes almost half the rate registered at the beginning of the 1990s, when it was 32‰. This does not alter the fact that in 2006 more than 5% of all deliveries in Poland were by women aged nineteen and younger, and the youngest mothers were twelve and thirteen year-old girls (in 2001 one mother was twelve, seven mothers were thirteen years-old[Malicka, 2003]). The decrease in the number of deliveries by teenagers applies more to women aged eighteen and nineteen, and less so to the youngest girls. The fertility of teenagers between the beginning of the 1990s and the year 2004 was as follows: among women aged nineteen, a decrease from 90‰ to 33‰ was registered, among eighteen year-old girls, a decrease from 50‰ to 21‰ was noted, among seventeen year-olds the rate decreased form 20‰ to 10‰, among sixteen year-old girls it decreased from 7‰ to 4‰, and for girls younger than sixteen year-old it decreased from 2 to 1.1‰ (Chazan, Gabryś, Środoń, Wróblewska 2007).

Table 3-1. The number of births by women aged nineteen or less, compared to the total number of births in Poland in the years 2003-2008 (only live births). Source: Rocznik Demograficzny, 2009.

Year	Total	Aged 19 and less	Percentage
2003	351 072	22 514	6.41%
2004	356 131	20 502	5.75%
2005	364 383	19 295	5.29%
2006	374 244	19 230	5.13%
2007	387 873	18 866	5.12%
2008	414 499	21 207	5.12%

The optimistic overtone of this data somehow subsides a little bit, when we take into account that the total number of all teenage girls in our country has decreased steadily since the mid-1990s, along with a decrease of the birth rate observed since 1984 and the period of population decline. Moreover, the data does not include the number of miscarriages and stillbirths that are observed in teenage girls much more often than in mature women (Hillis et al., 2004), nor does it include the number of abortions, since there is no data available concerning the scale of abortions in this group in Poland[3].

Negative consequences of teenage motherhood or earlier experienced abuse?

Both in foreign, and Polish literature, one finds much empirical data on the negative consequences of teenage motherhood. Among them are:

a) Health consequences for the mother and child, such as low birth weight, a higher risk of perinatal death when applied to the child and mother alike and a higher risk of infection with sexually transmitted diseases such as HIV/AIDS (Bidzan, 2007; Chazan, Gabryś, Środoń, Wróblewska, 2007; Hillis et al., 2004; Wróblewska 2002). Moreover, pregnancies of very young mothers are considered high risk pregnancies because of the immaturity of the uterus and other more frequent complications (Dębski 1999);
b) Socioeconomic consequences for the child's mother, including: interruption of education and the resulting lower level of education, difficulties in the course of career development, lower income and

economic problems (Bidzan, 2007; Chazan, Gabryś, Środoń, Wróblewska, 2007);

c) Demographic consequences, such as: single motherhood and marital failures as well as social burdens resulting from, for example, single-mother benefits (Boden, Fergusson, Horwood, 2008; Chazan, Gabryś, Środoń, Wróblewska, 2007).

This data is compatible with the stereotypic image of a teenage mother as a helpless person who "has ruined her life because of her mindlessness", turning into ashes her development and career. The question whether the premature pregnancy leads to the above-mentioned consequences, or is itself a consequence of social factors that affected her development earlier in her life, has been the subject of a lively debate in scientific literature for twenty years.

The latest studies verify theses about the cause and effect links between early motherhood and failures in life. New data show that just taking into account the variables preceding pregnancy and increasing the risk of pregnancy result in decreasing the gap between teenage mothers and those who have children later in life. For example, longitudinal studies conducted in New Zealand (Boden, Ferguson, Horwood, 2008), questioned statements about the relationship between early motherhood, higher degrees of mental disturbance, greater dependency on social services as well as lower levels of education, employment and earnings. The authors of the study pinpointed these factors to the family of origin of the teenage mother, and to the conditions she previously lived in (as well as to some other interfering variables), and not - directly - to teenage motherhood. Similarly, the study of Hillis et al. (2004) showed that the relationship between teenage motherhood and family, professional, financial and emotional difficulties occur exclusively in women who experienced some form of neglect or abuse in their childhood, but are not found among persons who grew up in adequately supportive environments.

Therefore, it appears that many adverse characteristics of the functioning of a mature person, ascribed to teenage pregnancy and the reality of assuming a maternal role prematurely, coincide with the characteristics of functioning typical for people who as children experienced abuse and neglect in their own family. What, then, are the links between violence and premature pregnancy?

The relationship between interpersonal violence and teenage motherhood - available data

Data on the links between the experiences of interpersonal violence and premature pregnancy that I am going to present come mainly from studies conducted in the United States, where the occurrence of teenage motherhood is much more frequent than it is in Poland[4]. The data covers both current abusive experiences and childhood experiences[5].

Abuse experienced by teenage girls who become mothers.

According to a report prepared in 2001 in the United States (Leiderman, Almo, 2001):

a) At least 25 percent of teenage mothers experienced interpersonal violence in the year when they became pregnant, mainly from their own partner, or possibly from other family members, and it comprised mainly verbal assaults, threats of physical assault, having objects thrown at them, face slapping, pushing, kicking, being threatened with a firearm, being threatened with having one used against them, intimidation, forced isolation, deprivation of all resources and forced sexual activity. In some studies this rate rises as high as 50 or even 80 percent;
b) Kellogg's (1999) studies prove that 13 percent of teenage pregnancies are a direct outcome of forced sexual intercourse;
c) Young women, especially teenagers who are pregnant or already mothers, are more vulnerable to interpersonal violence than older women. It could be stated that the younger the woman, the higher the risk of abuse in a close relationship: the risk is thirty to fifty percent higher in cases of younger teenagers when compared to women over twenty (Gessner, Perham-Hester 1998).

Unfortunately, in Poland there are no studies that provide an estimate of the extent of abuse experienced by teenage girls (including those who become pregnant) from their sexual partners. However, considering cultural factors and available data on domestic violence , one may suppose that the relationship between a teenager and her partner is also sometimes marked with violence[6], although estimating its scale requires empirical exploration.

Adverse childhood experiences of teenage mothers.

Interesting research on the links between adverse childhood experiences, teenage pregnancy, and disturbances in psychosocial functioning, was conducted in California by Susan Hillis and her collegues (2004) in the years 1995-1997. The study explored 9,159 women older than eighteen (mean age fifty-six), among whom twenty-three percent had become pregnant between ages eleven and nineteen. Among other factors, exposure to adverse childhood experiences was studied, including: emotional abuse, physical abuse, sexual abuse, and abuse between adult partners at home, living with an adult addicted to alcohol or drugs, living with a mentally ill adult, living with an adult with a criminal history, and divorce or separation of parents. Results showed that even the presence of just one of the above-mentioned experiences in the histories of women in the study increased the risk of teenage pregnancy by five percent, and each additional experience multiplied the rate of pregnancies so that it went up to fifty-six percent among those who reported all, or nearly all, of the adverse experiences, while only sixteen percent of women who did not report any adverse experiences became pregnant as teenagers. These results suggest that there is a cause and effect relationship between the experience of abuse or emotional/physical neglect, and the risk of becoming pregnant at a young age.

Though in Poland there are no studies examining the experiences of abuse or neglect preceding teenage pregnancy, the few available reports on small populations of teenage mothers show the presence of such problems in their nuclear families For example: parental alcoholism, unstable personal situation, domestic violence, lack of firm bonds, deprivation of emotional needs and neglect (Kościelska, 1998).

Sexual abuse in childhood and premature motherhood [7]

Most studies which aimed at verifying the thesis regarding a relationship between sexual abuse and premature pregnancy and motherhood confirmed these links, allowing one to postulate that many teenage mothers have experienced sexual abuse in their past. The studies cover many forms of this category of abuse, including sexual intercourse, and other sexually motivated behaviours, not necessarily resulting in physical contact. The links are confirmed both in longitudinal (Ferguson, Horwood, Lynskey, 1997) and in retrospective studies (Logan et al., 2007). For example, in a longitudinal study conducted for ten years (Noll, Tricket, Putnam, 2003), it was found that in a group of women abused sexually between the ages of six and sixteen by means of genital contact and/or penetration, eighty-two percent had a child as teenagers, compared to thirty-five percent of women from the control group. Moreover, the sexually abused women had their first babies at a significantly younger age than the controls. Similarly, other longitudinal studies (Fergusson, Horwood, Lynskey, 1997) and retrospective research show that there is a large number of teenage mothers among groups of women who were sexually abused as children (Landry, Forrest, 1995), and that this type of trauma among very young mothers is very frequent. Based on the above-cited report (Leiderman, Almo, 2001), it is assumed that thirty-three to sixty-six percent of teenage mothers at some point in their lives experienced sexual abuse.

It should be stressed that there exist some isolated reports questioning these theses (conf. Smith 1996; Widom, Kuhns, 1996; Witwer, 1997), and point to the role of other factors related to premature pregnancy, such as early sexual initiation, numerous partners, psychoactive substance abuse, poorly educated parents, and low level of aspirations and accomplishment. Nevertheless, it is known that some of these variables are linked to child sexual abuse; therefore they may play a mediatory role in the relationship between childhood trauma and premature motherhood.

It is also worth emphasizing that difficulties in reviewing the existing studies on the links between interpersonal violence and premature pregnancy is a result of differences in defining violence by various authors, who include under this heading a wider or narrower spectrum of these experiences, and use a variety of procedures and research tools. Therefore, although many studies show the relationship between the experience of interpersonal trauma and teenage motherhood, precise estimations of the extent of these links and descriptions of their nature is a task for the future. The same applies to the exploration of the problem in Poland, where it has never been subjected to empirical verification.

How does the experience of abuse lead to premature pregnancy?

According to studies conducted in the United States and other Western countries, there exist many complex links between the experience of interpersonal violence and premature motherhood. Generally speaking, the experience of violence may be related to premature pregnancy in two ways: directly and/or indirectly (Leiderman, Almo, 2001).

The link is direct when pregnancy is a result of forced sexual contact, leading to fertilization, or when it is an effect of sabotaging the use of birth control methods by the partner. It seems that teenage girls not only have no knowledge about birth control methods (conf. Bidzan 2007), but they are frequently discouraged from using them by their partners. Leiderman and Almo (2001) turn our attention to the attitudes of men that may explain their reluctance to use contraceptives by any of the partners. For example: "a woman who protects herself against pregnancy may be unfaithful", "a woman with a child will not walk away", "a woman is more attractive sexually when she is fertile" etc.

The link is indirect when abuse is related to premature motherhood by means of the influence it has on the broadly defined development of a girl (or woman), leading her to engage in behaviours, situations and relationships which increase the possibility of her becoming pregnant. The factors mediating between interpersonal violence (particularly of a sexual nature) and early pregnancy are considered in the following, interlocking contexts:

1. Early departure from the family home by a teenager: the experience of domestic violence may lead to flight from home and a resort to prostitution for a living or undertaking sexual activity in exchange for accommodation or board (Leiderman, Almo, 2001).

2 Psychoactive substance abuse and engaging in risk behaviours: girls who experience insufficient parental care, abuse or neglect are prone to reach for alcohol and drugs and engage in risk behaviours, which may increase the possibility of their becoming pregnant through casual sexual contacts (Leiderman, Almo, 2001).

3. Using birth control methods: women who suffered abuse definitely less frequently use contraceptives (Logan et al., 2007).

4. Trauma re-enactment and further victimization: experience of abuse (particularly sexual abuse) in childhood increases the likelihood of engaging in other relationships based on the same pattern in adolescence and adulthood, entailing a risk of submitting oneself to forced sexual activity and becoming the victim of rape (Leiderman, Almo, 2001; Logan et al., 2007; Noll, Trickett, Putnam, 2003).

5. The outcome of overly intense and premature sexual stimulation: sexual abuse may ensue in excessive preoccupation with this sphere of functioning and lead to early sexual initiation, sexual contacts with numerous partners, and a tendency to engage in sexual activity with much older men who are reluctant to use contraceptives (Boyer, Fineman, 1992; Logan et al., 2007; Noll, Trickett, Putnam, 2003).

6. Unfulfilled emotional needs and their compensation: every form of abuse or neglect leads to the frustration of an individual's emotional needs, which should be fulfilled in a secure relationship based on trust with an

adult (adults). This developmental deficit disrupts the process of building an adequate, integrated self-image, and usually causes low self-esteem (in cases of sexual abuse quite often built on sexual attractiveness). The consequence of this state of affairs may be, on one hand, engaging in sexual activity motivated by the urge to fulfill frustrated emotional needs (contact, security, acceptance) in a relationship with a partner, while on the other hand it may mean becoming pregnant intentionally or sub-intentionally in the hope (expressed directly by some girls) of compensating for experienced frustration in the relationship with their own child (Bidzan, 2007; Boyer, Fineman, 1992; Kościelska, 1998; Skowrońska, 2009). Simultaneously, an important need that emerges fully during adolescence is the need for autonomy which can also play its role in the early decision about motherhood. Becoming pregnant may be perceived by a teenager as serving her to free herself from pathogenic family relationships (Boyer, Fineman, 1992) or to emphasise her own independence and freedom to decide for herself (Kościelska, 1998; Skowrońska, 2009). It is interesting that some studies prove that sexually abused girls more frequently express the desire to become pregnant out of fear of infertility (Rainey, Stevens-Simon, Kaplan, 1995), motivating them to try to become pregnant. It is possible that for these young women, for whom - because of adverse developmental conditions - it was more difficult to create a positive self-image based on interpersonal relationships, school accomplishments or their own interests, motherhood becomes a chance to compensate for this deficit through activation of the basic ability inherent in all humans to have one's own offspring.

7. Trans-generational pattern of violence or sexual abuse and early reproduction: for teenagers who become mothers as a result of trauma, it is often difficult to satisfy the needs of their own children, both physically (as well as materially) and emotionally, since their competence in this respect is insufficient. Therefore, establishing a stable relationship with their child, based on adequate recognition and response to the child's needs, may be a challenge exceeding the capabilities of a teenage mother, and will potentially interfere with the child's development in such a way that repeating the pattern of early parenthood in the next generation will be its far-reaching consequence (Leiderman, Almo, 2001).

Even though most of the above-mechanisms mediating between childhood experiences of trauma and teenage motherhood have the status of hypotheses, they shed new light on the discussed phenomenon. It seems that at least those premature pregnancies that are perceived as a social problem (where the mother is left alone, forced to use institutional support, helpless and inefficient as a parent) may be and often are both a direct and indirect effect of a complex trauma.

Moreover, apart from the above-mentioned mediating mechanisms, attention is given to other factors accompanying both interpersonal violence, and early motherhood, such as: poverty, a low standard of living as culturally determined (and in some environments accepted), oppressive attitudes toward women and treatment of them as objects, particularly when they are members of national minorities or are very young (adolescent girls).

Summary

The above-analysis of data and hypotheses is not free from certain weak points. They result, first of all, from a variety of methodologies used by researchers who do not always refer to the same definitions of violence and employ different tools to explore the same variable. Second, in the majority of the cited studies, reports on abuse are treated as tentative estimations, assuming that people are often too ashamed or embarrassed to talk about the trauma they experienced. It is highly probable that in reality the occurrence of such experiences may be much higher than the empirical data shows. Third, the applicability of the conclusions drawn from the cited studies is limited because of a number of social, cultural and economic differences. It may be thought that in Poland (where the rate of girls becoming pregnant is definitely lower than it is in the United States), the phenomenon of teenage motherhood is modified by such variables as social norms, anchored in Catholicism, flourishing in our country, the law concerning abortion or childcare, and the quality of social services and institutional support potentially offered to juvenile parents.

Notwithstanding the above-mentioned limitations, the problem of links between interpersonal trauma and premature motherhood deserves our attention, particularly among professionals dealing with such young parents, and undoubtedly requires research in our country. As teenage mothers in Poland still encounter stigmas and humiliating comments from medical workers in the public health service, as well as labels by family members or peers (conf. Skowrońska, 2009) - there is still much to be done. Awareness of the complexity of the situation that a young woman can find herself in, as well as understanding the psychological and social mechanisms mediating the trauma and experience of premature motherhood, gives hope to teenage mothers for accurate therapeutic and preventive interventions, thus helping them to avoid secondary victimisation in their already sorely tried lives.

In closing, I would like to express my own thought that teenage motherhood, when it is a direct or distant result of experienced violence, however hard it is, does not have to reduce chances for life success for the mother, or for the baby she is raising. For this to happen, aid activities (formal and informal) are necessary, allowing the young mother to build up her emotional and social competencies, as well as to overcome the limitations of past - often painful - experiences.

Notes

[1] Sexual education under the heading of "upbringing for the life in the family" has not been complying in this respect with international standards for many years (Polish Federation for Women and Family Planning, 2008), which has contributed to the consolidation of activities of many nongovernmental organizations aimed at promoting sexual education within the framework of "The agreement for the promotion of sexual education of children and teenagers in Polish schools" ratified in January 2009. The agreement is supported by the authority of such scholars as Prof. Zbigniew Izdebski, Prof. Zbigniew Lew Starowicz, Prof. Stanisław Obirek and Prof. Magdalena Środa (Polish Federation for Women and Family Planning, 2009).

[2] Stanisław Nastaj, vice-chairman of the Council of Pulawy County and a member of PiS (Law and Justice - Polish conservative political party), became infamous in September 2009 for his statement that pregnant students "should be isolated" because of their "bad example" to other girls and because "they themselves feel bad around others and others feel bad around them" (Iwon, 2009).

[3] According to a report on the implementation of "Family Planning, Preservation of the Human Foetus, and the Conditions of Admissibility for Abortion, and the Consequences of its Performance Act" in Poland in the years 2002-2007, there were 159, 174, 193, 225, 340 and 322 abortions performed respectively during those years (Rada Ministrów RP, 2009). It must be added, however, that this data is considered underestimated, and not reflecting the actual number of abortions performed (conf. Nowicka, 2007).

[4] In the United States, there were 66.2 pregnancies (terminated by abortion or ending in childbirth) for one thousand teenagers in 2002, which is thirty percent less than in 1990 (McKay 2006). This decrease may be explained in part by prevention programs implemented by numerous organizations appointed for this purpose.

[5] Not all studies differentiate between these two chronologically various experiences. Simultaneously, it is worth noting that in case of teenage mothers - particularly the younger ones - adverse childhood experiences often overlap and create a picture of abuse experienced by the girl ; therefore it is often impossible to draw a line between them.

[6] Estimating the scale of domestic violence in Poland is a difficult task- women and children, for cultural, economic and psychological reasons, often conceal the

fact of being abused by their loved ones. It is estimated that eighteen to fifty-one percent of women in Poland experience domestic violence, and that governmental preventive and remedial programs are considered inconsistent and absolutely ineffective in counteracting this phenomenon in the long run (Nowakowska, Jabłońska, 2003).

[7] One difficulty in summarizing this study results from the fact that various authors include various experiences, and thus sexual abuse may be considered to be: rape or attempted rape, forced sexual acts, sexual contact with an adult, or events considered by the respondents as sexual abuse or any type of sexual touch (Logan, Holcombe, Ryan, Manlove, Moore 2007).

CHAPTER FOUR

THE LIFE ACTIVITY OF WOMEN-VICTIMS OF DOMESTIC VIOLENCE AS A DETERMINANT OF VICTIMISATION SUSCEPTIBILITY

IRENA POSPISZYL

Literature and public opinion on the topic of women as victims of domestic violence offer extensive proof that the most apt predictor of all sorts of recurring harm is its past experiencing. By way of example, Brunon Hołyst (1999) asserted that in those instances when a given person had been the victim of rape at least upon a single occasion the probability of undergoing such an act of violence again is 3,8 times greater then in the case of those persons who had never experienced it previously. The same holds true for victims of childhood sexual abuse, violence, theft or similar felonies (cf. Roy M. 1977:Walker L.1988 : Breslau, N. Davis G. C. Andreski P. Peterson E. L. Schulz L. 1997: Pospiszyl I. 1994, 2003: Messman T. L., Long P. J., 1996: Wilkin A. 1998: Brown K.,1999: Lis-Turlejska M. 2002: et al.). Numerous hypotheses attempt to explain the reasons for the chronic nature of experiencing harm, starting with the simplest reasons such as gender, age, the attractive appearance of the victim, and her provocative behaviour or absentmindedness, to multi-factor personality analyses or the negative consequences of the trauma. Mathematical hypotheses such as the one proposed by Prof. Doliński maintain that victimisation susceptibility can be deduced upon the basis of a probability calculus, which maintains that if certain crimes are committed by the same person upon numerous occasions then the number of victims is multiple and the situation of the victim and the perpetrator must recur.

In the case of victims of violence, the most popular thesis explaining victimisation susceptibility is the conviction, to different degrees confirmed by research, that experiencing violence in the past somehow deprives the individual of the ability to protect herself against a similar experience in the future (Walker L. 1988:Herman L. H.1998: Brown H. 1999,:Seligmann M. E. 1974, 1993). If we were to add such intervening variables as gender or the type of used defensive mechanisms. then it would appear that we have at our disposal a compendium of knowledge about an individual's susceptibility to turn into a victim of violence.

Research objective

Despite the outright obvious conclusions about victimisation susceptibility being the outcome of experienced traumas, the existing situation is neither unambiguous nor even satisfactory. If we were to accept that victims of violence have developed a certain *learned helplessness,* which makes it difficult for them to protect themselves against re-victimisation and, as a result, encompasses other domains of life, then we assume that prior to those experiences such victims were not helpless in the face of the assorted events that occurred in their lives, and that they have created such helplessness. This helplessness manifested as passivity when they are convicted based only upon an experienced violence rendered permanent in their consciousness, that resistance will be ineffective.

The heart of the matter lies in the fact that such conclusions are drawn *post factum*, i.e. already while examining the victims of violence frequently chronic victims of violence and accepting *implicite* that they are the consequences of violence. On the other hand, little is known about the way in which those victims functioned prior to confronting a traumatic situation, how they tackled other social situations and whether they had not revealed this particular passivity already in the past. The topic of the analysis presented below will involve answering the above-posed questions. Naturally, it is difficult to ascertain exactly how the victims dealt with difficult situations in the past, before they experienced violence, since they do not have to remember this and therefore assess their past experiences *via* the present-day situation (by mixing up facts, projecting emotions, etc.). Finally, they could compensate their difficult experiences by idealising the past. On the other hand, one could take a closer look at the past of the examined women without referring to their traumatic experiences, see how they functioned in spheres not connected with traumatic experiences, and analyse their life dynamism before they became victims.

Method

While embarking upon answers to the earlier formulated questions, research has resorted to a modified version of the life activity questionnaire constructed by the author in the 1980s and adapted to contemporary conditions. The questionnaire is composed of 36 questions (open and closed) pertaining to four spheres of the activeness of the examined individuals. The first focuses on childhood social activity, with particular attention paid to the school period. The second concerns the professional activity of the adult. The next sphere encompasses the social activity of the adult, and the fourth relates to the family situation. All responses were based on the declarations made by the examined women concerning their activeness. Furthermore, the questionnaire included additional questions about the forms of the violence experienced in the past. Persons from the control group who answered questions about physical violence in the affirmative were excluded from further analysis.

The analysis presented below involves two groups, each composed of a hundred grownup women. The first the experimental group, includes victims of violence perpetrated by their partners. The study took into consideration only women in a steady relationship for a minimum of three years, and who had been the victims of physical violence at least upon several occasions. The second, the control group, was composed of women who declared that they had never experienced physical violence committed by their partner. The control group had been chosen deliberately, also from the viewpoint of education, place of residence and duration of the relationship. Whenever it was possible, the questionnaire tried to take into account persons similar to the experimental group as regards the listed criteria. The research was conducted for several years in Warsaw and its environs. As a rule, the women were recruited through the intermediary of detox clinics, crisis intervention centers, social help centers and therapy support groups intended for the victims of violence.

The average age of the women in the experimental group was 43 in the control group 38. The youngest member of the experimental group was 27 and the oldest 62. As a rule, the women belonged to the 35-50 age group. The youngest representative of the control group was 23 and the oldest54. The largest number was composed of women older than 35. In both groups the percentage of women older than 35 was 64%.

The average relationship lasted for 10-20 years. Precise data are presented in Table 4-1.

Table 4-1 Relationship duration - %

Relationship duration	Violence victims	Non-victims
up to 5 years	10	13
5-10 years	3	11
10-20 years	50	43
more than 20 years	37	33

Evidently, the majority of the examined women found themselves at an age of stability or relative stability, described by certain family experts as the stereotypy phase (cf. Baker 1984).

Results

An analysis of the results comprises an element of a larger project of research on the victimological susceptibility of the victims of violence, conducted by the author for many years. As is known, an important element of an individual's independence and social activity is his/her education and professional activity. This is the reason why this particular question was taken into account as prime in the examined groups of women. Vocational and secondary education dominates.

Table 4 -2 Education

Education	Violence victims %	Non-victims %
primary	10	7
vocational	24	29
secondary	58	54
Higher	8	11

The education of the examined women is not subjected to a comparative analysis since the control group had been chosen deliberately by taking into consideration the similarity of education, so that such features as age, education, and place of residence or, finally, the duration of the relationship would be relatively uniform. (Taking into account so many criteria simultaneously makes it difficult to select groups that would be ideal from the viewpoint of demographic traits; this would entail arranging them in pairs. Such a process would be lengthy and, in the opinion of the author, would not alter much as regards the ultimate results). It is important to compare similar phases in the life of the examined women in the compared groups.

The majority of the women in question are professionally active, although the percentage of non-working women is also relatively large. In the experimental group professionally active women comprise 78% (including four retired). The group of non-victims of violence includes 68% professionally active women, i.e., a slightly smaller number. The author found these data surprising, since usually pertinent literature claims that female victims of violence are, generally speaking, financially more dependent on their partners.

An important factor modifying the life activity of the women is the number of dependent children. By way of example, the professional activity and social mobility of women with three children or more are decidedly less than those of women with a single child or who are childless. In the examined sample, the number of children corresponds to the normal distribution.

Table 4-3 Number of children

Number of children	Violence victims	Non-victims
Childless	13	10
One child	41	53
Two children	32	33
Three and more children	10	7

As a rule, the women have one or two children. The studied samples contain a slightly smaller number of childless women than is the case in the whole population, but this probably stems from the fact that the women were chosen deliberately. Let us recall that one of the criteria was remaining in a relationship.

Women-victims of violence were additionally asked to assess the reasons for the partner's resort to violence and were permitted to indicate more than a single cause. The decisive majority mentioned alcohol abuse - 78%. Moreover, many women spoke about their partner's "character", "nature" and "personality" - 37 %, assorted problems with which the partner is incapable of dealing - 32 % (involving work, life, health, family, children), upbringing - 27% ("this is the way he had been brought up", "his father and brothers are the same") and mental disorders - 12% ("he is abnormal"); finally, 4% were unable to point out any reasons. Despite the great variety of the indications it is amazing to see just how many women seek the reasons for their partner's aggression in his problems and weaknesses and not in their own feature character traits and provocation, as some of the authors describing the victims would have it. Apparently, such women make relatively realistic assessments concerning the direct causes of violence.

One of the key variables was the evaluation of the expansiveness of the women during childhood and adolescence. The studies took into consideration participation in circles, sports and social activity, the number of friends and the frequency of meetings with peers. They also registered each indication of the examined women without a detailed analysis of the degree of advancement in a given discipline, including such indices as: participation in science and art circles (biology, chemistry, the protection of the natural environment, geography), sports clubs, the pursuit of a certain domain of the arts (e.g. music), regular participation in sports (e.g. netball), voluntary work, activity in clubs, teams, associations or church organisations. Social activity was also measured by participation in social campaigns, for instance, those conducted for the sake of the protection of the natural environment, charity work or discussion clubs. In turn, social life was measured by the frequency of meetings with friends and the number of the latter. The analysis pertains exclusively to the frequency of indications pertaining to different forms of activity, without delving into the degree of advancement in the particular forms of such activity. It was recognised that the questions are sufficiently neutral not to set into motion the need for social approval. Even when the examined women slightly exaggerated, this too can testify to their positive attitude towards such activity.

The outcome of the examination of social activity revealed a rather interesting tendency. In an overwhelming majority of the analysed indicators the victims of violence revealed small, less childhood activity than women who do did not experience violence in their relationships. Not always did it such activity attain the level of statistical active feasibility, but almost all indices revealed a conspicuous tendency. Generally speaking, women-victims of violence had been more passive in their past than those women who were not subjected to violence (exact data is presented in Table 4-4).

Table 4-4 Social activity of women-victims of violence in their past - significant differences

Women's activity in the past	Women violence victims N=100		Women non-victims N=100		t	p
	X	s.d.	X	s.d.		
Participation in interest circles	0.91	2.48	1.22	3.12	6.12	.0001
Sport	0.78	0.67	0.94	0.87	1.70	n.i
Social life	1.97	1.01	2.04	1.14	3.50	.001
Social activity	0.68	1.28	0.72	0.97	3.22	.001
Leadership experience	0.56	0.66	0.52	0.63	1.10	n.i

s.d. - standard deviation
n.i. - statistically insignificant

These women did not take such a large part in interest circles, had fewer friends, were more rarely involved in social activity and, finally, were less interested in sport, although in the last case one can detect only a tendency, since its research results had not attained the level of statistical significance. Statistically significant differences also did not occur as regards leadership experiences. A certain predominance of women-victims was, however, distinct. (The researchers requested the women to say how many times they had acted as school prefects, leaders of a sports group, in the Scout movement, at a camp, in an ensemble or a social campaign). The respondents were permitted to mention everything that they regarded as leading others.

Generally speaking, the greater passivity of the women-victims in the light of the above-mentioned indices could point to the fact that from the very onset they possessed a smaller predisposition for dealing with the social world (and, unquestionably, pertinent experiences).

The presented research also brings to mind a certain general reflection, namely, that the social activity of all the examined women does not appear to be expansive. On the average, the women took part in less than a single circle, there were some who had not been engaged in sports of any kind, and in school never became involved in any sort of social activity. Naturally, statistical knowledge tends to distort the results. In certain cases, some respondents had been very active as children, while others had little to boast of. The average, however, shows that even active women were scarce.

Things are not quite so obvious as regards the life activeness of adult women. Apparently, battered women worked more frequently, and thus were professionally more active. Such professional activity constitutes not only a prominent element of social activity but is also an essential source of the woman's financial independence, a factor that is treated as a relevant predictor of liberating oneself from a destructive relationship.

As has been noted, the objective of the research was to assess the life dynamism of women upon the basis of various spheres of social activity; this is the reason why the respondents were asked to mention the sort of social activeness in which they took part in the past ten years. In order to facilitate the answers, the questionnaire contains several proposals of responses, and the women were asked to add answers that had not been suggested. The questionnaire took into account the following forms of activity:

1. Activity in political parties, clubs and organisations, associations, foundations and circles (scientific, tourist, sport, social, art, etc.)
2. Activity in educational institutions attended by the children (PTA, etc.)
3. Involvement in neighbourhood and housing estate activity and work conducted for the sake of the closest surrounding (in housing estate councils, for the sake of the protection of the natural environment, the protection of animals, etc.)
4. Activity in social and art clubs and societies (e.g. fan clubs).
5. Participation in social campaigns, demonstrations and programmes.

By way of example: campaigns associated with the protection of the natural environment (cleaning up the world), pro-health (a day without a cigarette), civic (equal rights parades), pro-community (building a new road), the workplace (safety first). The above are only examples of assorted forms of involvement that the women could list. In these cases too, the researchers were interested not only in the sort of activeness but also in the fact of its initiation and the frequency of participation. The examined women could mention all the campaigns and groups in which they had participated. It is worth adding that the studies had intentionally ignored social life activity connected with the family since such activity is often delineated by a certain family tradition and the pressure exerted by its closest surroundings, entailing meetings and contacts. The authors of the questionnaire were concerned with such forms of activity that suggested a greater probability that the persons under examination had initiated them.

The obtained results also confirm earlier findings, namely, that generally speaking the activity of women is relatively low and the number of victims even lower. Precise data are to be found in Table 4-5.

Table 4-5. Social activity of women-victims of violence as adults

Forms of activity	Victims %	Non-victims %
Activity in political parties, clubs, organisations	2	4
Activity in associations, foundations, circles	5	4
Activity in educational institutions attended by children	23	47
Involvement in neighbourhood, housing estate, etc.	15	19
Activity in social or art clubs and societies	11	18
Activity in social campaigns	31	41
Others (Church)	23	11

It is not surprising that women most often take part in activeness linked with their children's school life and social campaigns that frequently possess an incidental character stimulated by the mass media or social community requirements. Although the qualitative analysis notices a certain predominance of women who do not experience violence, the differences do not appear to be conspicuous; hence the use of the Student's-t test in order to determine whether such differences actually do occur and, if so, on what level. The average was calculated on the basis of the indications of participation in assorted social campaigns. The results proved to be rather startling.

Table 4-6. Significant differences between averages concerning the social activity of women-victims of violence and women who are not victims of domestic violence

Groups	x	s.d.	t	P
Violence victims	1.11	9.60	12.93	.00000
Non-victims	1.44	11.50		

The significance of differences between the compared groups turned out to be extremely high. Women who are not the victims of violence take part in assorted social campaigns much more frequently; the same holds true for activity associated with the education of their children, the neighbourhood and social life. The only form of social activity that involves the victims of violence more often is linked with the religious community; their presence in associations and foundations is slightly more frequent. Emphasis is due to the fact that women-members of both examined groups revealed only slight interest in religious organisations.

Conclusions

The obtained results of research focusing on the life activity of women-victims of violence are rather unambiguous. The research premises were based on a somewhat universal conviction, frequently corroborated by experimental and anamnestic studies, that due to experienced violence female victims develop a feeling of helplessness towards their life a passivity and generally weak ability to act for the sake of altering their situation. This explain why women -victims remain in a destructive relationship, exhibit relatively slight activity intent on changing their life situation, show a dependence upon the partner and even demonstrate an inclination towards addiction.

This study decided to verify the above-findings, albeit in slightly a different manner. The author referred to forms of the life activity of women-victims of violence other than family relations, and to examine their life dynamism both as adolescents and adults. At the same time, unconcerned with a precise determination of the interests and activities of the women under examination, the author was interested in studying their readiness to undertake such activity, the need to be active and involve themselves in assorted spheres of life, to realize their interests, and to develop a *sui generis* life driving force realised in various domains of activeness, which, as it had been assumed *implicite*, can become useful also in an oppressive situation. Such an approach appears to be a good point of reference for later experiences, in this case traumatic, is relatively easy to examine and rarely susceptible to falsehoods associated with the time risk.

The obtained outcome of the research disclosed interesting conclusions.

1. Women-victims of violence disclosed a generally greater passivity in social life, both during childhood and as adults. Significantly, this passivity was demonstrated in the majority of the measured features.
2. Despite the generally greater life passivity of the women-victims of violence as compared to women without such experiences, in certain spheres of life members of the basic group revealed higher professional activity on a statistically significant level. Their more frequent life activity makes it possible to assume that financial dependency is not a circumstance that explains remaining in a destructive situation. It must be added, however, that to a great degree this is the result of the specificity of Polish conditions. Access to adult victims of violence in Poland is associated with the partner's alcohol addiction: addiction therapy centres make it easier to reach adult victims of violence. In turn, the partner's addiction frequently makes it necessary for the woman to take over the burden of providing subsistence for the family and thus to go to work. Professional activity could be, therefore, imposed by additional circumstances.
3. No differences were discovered between the compared groups of women as regards the number of children, a factor frequently pointed out as the reason for women's greater dependence upon their partners.

Summing up, the above studies have shown that the greater life passivity of women-victims of violence can be a relevant factor in explaining the victimological susceptibility of adult women-victims of violence. Despite the fact that such victims are rather active professionally, a situation probably enforced by living with an often addicted partner and the ensuing necessity of providing subsistence for the family, they are socially more isolated and less concentrated on other domains of social life, which could comprise not only a form of compensation for family problems but, additionally, make it easier to find help against violence. Finally, another significant element is social control connected with participation in social life. One cannot exclude the possibility that women would already be better protected against violence already by the very fact of a greater presence of other people in their lives.

CHAPTER FIVE

PARENT-CHILD ATTACHMENT AND PARTNER RELATIONSHIPS FORMED BY PERSONS AFTER CHILDHOOD TRAUMA

AGNIESZKA WIDERA-WYSOCZAŃSKA

Research results presented in this article concern the consequences of dysfunctional mother-child attachments and the complex, interpersonal childhood trauma evident in adult life in forming relations with a partner.

According to Mary Salter Ainsworth (1993), childhood attachment determines our life us much as biological factors, genetic constitution, cultural influences and individual experiences do. The most important is of course the bond between mother - or her surrogate in the case of her temporal or permanent absence - and child. Radke-Yarrow (1993) maintain that the bond of mother to kid is the core component in the care-giving system. In healthy mother-child relationships, mothers, who are confident in themselves, react sensitively, responsively and adequately to their children's emotional, cognitive or social needs. Attachment between mother and child is responsible for shaping the success or failure of future intimate relationships, the ability to maintain emotional balance, the ability to enjoy being ourselves and to find satisfaction in being with others, the ability to rebound from disappointment, discouragement, and misfortune, and to develop meaningful connections with others (Radke-Yarrow, 1993; Parkes, Stevenson-Hinde, Morris, 1993).

Therefore it is interesting to note what happens when mothers are abusive. What kinds of environments do they create for their children and what are the psychosocial consequences for the children in their future? Translation of emotional, physical, sexual violence or alcoholism into the mother's role of, suggests problems for the mother-child relationship, child development and its later adult life. The question arises whether and how the childhood attachment bond influences the quality and development of relationships in adult life. The answer should show us to what extent our adult decisions and reactions are influenced by childhood experiences. Numerous arguments in literature provide us with answers. Weiss (1993) points out that properties of childhood attachment and adult attachment are the same. The same because of the merging of emotions, motivations, possibilities of attention, and energy concentration. But different because of dissimilar expectations that the attachment figure has.

We are dealing with the same emotional system but whose perceptual elements have been modified. It's also interesting to note how the attachment system from childhood influences the choice of an adult relational figure. The determinants of mate selection has been much debated (Weiss, 1993). According to some theories, attachment from childhood is of no consequence to the choice of a partner unlike the mutual attraction, similar values, interests and goals. Others claim that early attachment experience decides most easily the kinds of partners with whom new attachments, as well as the developmental course of such new attachments, are formed .

Stith, Rosen, Middleton, Busch, Lundeberg and Carlton (2000), based on the meta-analysis of numerous published research results, proved that witnessing or experiencing violence in childhood encourages involvement in building marital relations based on violence. Walker, Logan and Jordan (2004) connected research on childhood and the quality of intimate relationships with a partner, with further consequences such as separation and divorce and the influence of these traumatic experiences on the life of the conflicted partners' children.

The research results presented here describe findings that emerged from a large study that explored risk factors encouraging violence in the family and thus causing its intergenerational transfer. The purpose of that part of the study was to discover links between the type of abuse experienced, type of mother-child attachment in childhood, and the quality of relationships with the partner in adulthood (Figure 5-1).

Figure 5-1. Research diagram

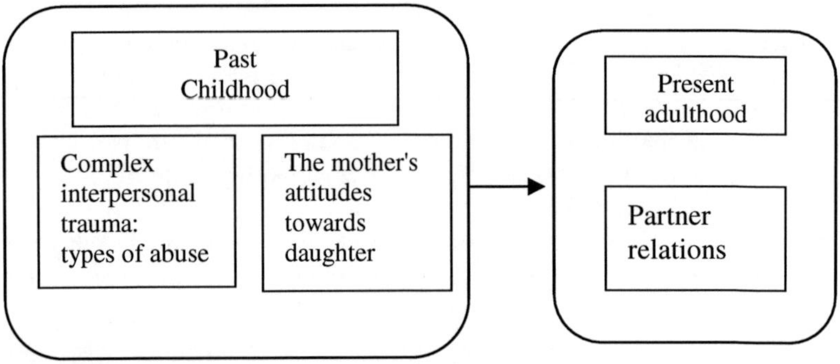

The following questions were asked: what kind of mothers' approach to their daughters can be specified in violence-afflicted families? What type of partner was chosen by such a mother's daughter in her adult life? What are these partners' characteristics and what sort of relationship is built up between them?

Understanding of attachment and family violence

Interpretations of some terms useful for this article are presented below. In order to emphasize the unique nature of the attachment phenomenon [(from others relational) , literature employs certain qualities: 1. proximity seeking, when the child attempts to remain within protective range of its parents; 2. secure based effect, when the presence of an attachment figure fosters security in the child and as a result encourages confident exploration and play, and communication with the mother teaches it to make plans, goals and choices; 3. separation protest, when threat to the continued accessibility of the attachment figure gives rise to protest and to active attempts to ward off the separation; 4. specificity of attachment figure, because once attachment to a particular figure has been formed, only that figure is an object of attachment and gives security, while separation from the figure gives rise to protest. Attempts to substitute another figure fails, no matter how solicitous or caring the other figure may be; and 5. insensitivity of experience with the attachment figure, because attachment seems to persist even when the attachment figure is neglecting or abusive (Parkes, Stevenson-Hinde, Morris, 1993; Weiss, 1993; Cassidy, Shaver, 1999; Rich, 2006).

Complex interpersonal, psychological trauma means a repeated, traumatic, chronic complex and interpersonal experience - caused by action of a close person. To this category belong various kinds of neglect and violence experienced since early childhood, through periods crucial for development - often adolescence - until the present moment of their life and their forming a new relationship. It causes all kinds of symptoms visible in all life spheres: emotional, cognitive, social, intimate, connected with the partner or family, somatic, and spiritual. The nature of the symptoms changes within the life-span. It can result in their accumulation and development of secondary life problems, including interpersonal ones. In case of particularly severe trauma, these symptoms can lead to serious mental disorders (Terr, 1994; Allen, 2001).

Emotional trauma (abuse), includes all humiliating attitudes, or behaviors intended to diminish a child's (or other person's) sense of worth and which disturb its sense of life. During the study the following types of behavior by a parent or other caretaker were considered: neglect, rejection (abandonment), degradation (criticism, name-calling), terrorization (screaming/shouting), emotional isolation (silence, no talks), corruption, exploitation (demands which surpass the child's abilities), denial, and inconsistent parenting (Briere, 1992). Physical trauma (abuse) consists of an adult's behavior directed towards a child's (or other person's, e.g. the mother's, fathers', siblings') body, the results of which may, or does, constitute physical injury. Active physical abuse (for example: various forms of beating, forcing the person to perform denigrating tasks, and extremely brutal behavior, such as scalding, choking or inflicting cut wounds) as well as passive (e.g. prohibiting speaking, walking, or relieving one's physiological needs) were distinguished. Alcohol-related abuse consists of a wide array of chaotic and violent behaviors and attitudes concentrated around the use of alcohol or other psychoactive substances, or resulting from their use. Among these behaviors is disruption of the family structure, for example, the family's culture, rituals, bonds, parenting rules, and forcing dysfunctional roles upon the children.

Childhood Sexual Abuse was defined as sexual activity, which includes attitudes, beliefs, roles, and relations, as well as emotions, behaviors, words, and states, by means of which a dependent, immature child or adolescent, unable to express conscious, informed consent, who requires the unconditional protection of older persons (legally in Poland to the 15th year, in my opinion psychologically to the 18th year of age), as well as a person at any age is exploited by an older person or a peer to satisfy the perpetrator's needs involving, among others, feelings of strength, power, self-esteem, and sexual pleasure. To classify the sexual behaviors which represent an offence against a child (and other persons), I have differentiated groups of sexual abuse (Widera-Wysoczańska, 2007, 2010). The first group is called intra-familial sexual abuse, when the perpetrator is a direct caregiver of the child (e.g. father, mother, grandfather, grandmother) and/or other family member. The incest occurring here is described as biological, when there is contact between a perpetrator and a person with whom they have a close blood relationship (according to legal definitions) and he/she is a legal caregiver of the child (biological, adoptive, foster parents, grandparents, siblings. The second group is called extra-familial sexual abuse: the perpetrator is a person from outside the family, either known to the child (e.g. teacher, schoolmate, playmate, family friend) or a stranger. Psychological incest can occur here when the perpetrator is a person of authority for the child, a person whom the child trusts and expects interest and safety, and depends on him in some spheres of life (family friend, neighbor, teacher, etc.). Both groups include direct and indirect sexual abuse. Direct sexual abuse contains various types of actions: a. sexual abuse with touching including: touching, kissing, or fondling a child's intimate places, penetration of the child's sexual organs, forcing the child to intercourse and rape, masturbation in the presence of the child or forcing the child to do it for the perpetrator, conducting unnecessary medical or care procedures, using the child to produce pornographic pictures and films, bathing the child in such a way that it finds intrusive (touching the breasts and buttocks, often with vulgar remarks, of a maturing girl or other body parts, often in the presence of other family members); b. Sexual abuse without direct touching of the child (e.g. showing pornography, peeping, exposing oneself, having intercourse in the child's presence); c. Emotional sexual abuse (e.g. vulgar insults, role change, demands, the child becomes a parent's partner). Indirect sexual violence can be divided into a. bringing the child to the perpetrator; b. consciously allowing the child to be harmed; c. Not reacting to the sexual abuse of the child when the caregiver knows of it.

Methodology

In order to obtain deepened understanding of the phenomenon under investigation, psychological qualitative study was employed. The study included the women's retrospective, subjective consideration of their childhood, with special attention to abuse experienced then and the mothers' parental attitudes and relations with the partner as they were before beginning of the therapy. The talks took place at the beginning of the therapeutic process (during the first three individual sessions) and also after a year of group therapy.

Participants

The participants in the study were selected by criterion-based purposeful sampling (Patton, 1990). The sampling criteria to select the women were that participants (1) were in a relation with a partner at least two years; (2) they had experienced childhood abuse; (3) they had at least secondary education; (4) are able to retrospective and subjective perception of their childhood experience and also (3) these women were taking part in individual and group therapy for adult persons from dysfunctional families (the family of origin). They were recruited from different therapeutical groups for people who experienced childhood trauma.

Table 5-1. Demographic data: n=88; mean age: 31 years

Feature		N	%
Education	Higher	77	87.5
	Secondary	11	12.5
Marital status	in a marital relationship	38	43
	cohabiting	50	56.8

Eighty-eight female victims of complex chronic childhood abuse were between 21 and 44 years of age with a mean of 31 years. In terms of level of education, 77 (87.5%) persons had higher and 11 (12.5%) persons had secondary education. Thirty-eight women (43%) living in a marital situation while the rest were cohabiting for two years at least. (Tab. 5-1).

Research methods

The structured interviews "Family Childhood Abuse Questionnaire" and "Intimate Situations Questionnaire" were used to determine the type of childhood abuse experienced by the women. The structured interview "Retrospective Perception of Parental Attitudes" was used to identify the women's retrospective and subjective perception of their parents' (mother's) parental attitudes. The quality of intimate relationships in adulthood was investigated using the "Intimate Relationships" structured interview. The aforementioned research methods have been created for a multistage study on family-violence risk factors according to the rules of qualitative and quantitative method-making The questions included have been based on literature, the present researcher's practical knowledge, and numerous pilot studies as well as with the help of competent judges who added important qualifications to questions in their appropriate groups.

An open qualitative interview "Family Childhood Abuse Questionnaire" was used to obtain information about various types of violence (emotional, physical, sexual, addictions) in the family of origin, about its roles, rules, beliefs and relationships between members, , and about its structure. The structured, qualitative "Intimate Situations Questionnaire" (ISQ) provided information abort three types of direct and indirect sexual violence (described above) ,their length of time, and frequency.

"Retrospective Perception of Parental Attitudes" (RPPA) made it possible to recognize subjective perceptions by the examined women of their mothers' and fathers' behavior. The questionnaire contains 57 statements consisting of four dimensions of parental experiences: I - care and support versus blame and neglect, II - meeting a child's needs, III -

respecting boundaries, rules, and roles, and IV - feeling self-confident as both a parent and a partner in childrearing (detailed description below). The same questions are placed on the two scales concerning, separately, the mothers' and fathers' behavior. For the answers, a four-grade Likert's scale was used. The study was carried out in several stages including a qualitative reformulating of the questions, a test on content-accuracy using competent judges methods, a test of diagnostic accuracy of the questions - the choice of discriminative variable values was performed by a reliability test, a coherence test (compatibility, convergence, consistence) of inner dimensions, a reliability test of the RSZR questionnaire for both scales, and confirmative factor analysis. Evaluation of the judge conformity in respect to diagnostic accuracy of questions for each item was tested by variation value; interpretation of evaluation conformity was verified by Friedman's test. The Alfa Cronbacha in the heterogenic group is accordingly 0.958 on the mothers' behavior scale (n=704) and 0.952 for the fathers' behavior scale (n=474). The RMSEA for the "mother" scale is 0.045, for the "father" 0.044 (Widera-Wysoczańska, 2006, 2010, 2010a). A detailed description of the questionnaire's structure and some of the research results presented below are included in a book (being edited out), which also contains the author's own research on sexual-violence risk factors in the family (Widera-Wysoczańska, 2010b). Results of this questionnaire concerning their mothers' behavior were worked out qualitatively in the presented study.

The intimate relationship with the partner was evaluated using "Intimate Relationships". People tested in writing answered questions concerning their partner's behavior, their own feelings, thoughts and opinions about the relationship, and the relationship's characteristics. The interview also contains questions concerning the mother's and father's behavior in the childhood of the examined person, and how this person perceives the importance of parental behavior in forming her adult relationship with a partner.

Dimensions of parenting

Material on mother's behavior obtained from the study participants was analyzed and interpreted using four dimensions of parenting created before. These dimensions were created on the basis of pilot studies, literature analysis, clinical experience, and discussions with specialists in the given field, statistical research and with the help of competent judges (Widera-Wysoczańska, 2010, 2010a).

The first dimension concerns "care and support vs. neglect and accusation". Problems are connected with the quality of basic care (accommodation, clothing, food, and neglect of basic care) and emotional aspects; with the quality of support and care given in difficult and pleasant circumstances (care, affection, emotional warmth, empathy, closeness and emotional coldness, rejection); ways of justifying the destructive behavior of the other parent; the quality of protection against physical, sexual or emotional threats (not employing abuse, protection against physical, sexual or emotional threats or employing abuse, exposing the child to abuse by other persons, lack of protection from other perpetrators); questions of methods of resolving family conflicts (constructive methods or not resolving conflict).

The second dimension called "Quality level of fulfilling the child's needs" describes the level of openness, recognition and adequate reaction to a child's needs (the caregiver knows and meets the child's needs or does not recognize or fulfill the child's needs, allows the child to satisfy its own needs or knows but does not fulfill the child's needs, indifference, lack of interest),and the control level over it (overprotection, intrusion, excessive contact and prevention, independent behavior) its emotions, feelings, interests or problems (allows the child to express feelings about itself, allows the child to express feelings to the parents, is interested in the child's, feelings, and problems, does not permit the child to express feelings, also to the parents).

The third dimension, "Quality of respecting boundaries, rules, and roles", describes problems with flexible or rigid, agreed or enforced boundaries in the family, their adaptation to circumstances; respecting enforced or agreed rules, the level of adequateness in enforcing and accepting roles in the family suitable to the age, developmental level, and person's status in the family; fulfilling parental needs with the aid of the child; suitability of rewards and punishments in given circumstances.

The fourth dimension concerns the "quality of self-assurance as a parent and partner in childrearing". It describes the level of satisfaction and happiness of being a parent, or feeling insecure or dissatisfied in being a parent measured with the ability (or the lack of it) of self-criticism; the ability to admit mistakes, apologize to the child; showing the child love, suitable or unsuitable ways of expressing various feelings to a child, demanding unconditional respect, lack of control over the parents' own reactions (e.g. inappropriate aggression); authoritarianism, despotism, control; level of complaint or satisfaction about being a parent (aversion to one's own parenting and to the child); quality of support in the marriage with respect to shared responsibility in childrearing or slandering each other.

Procedure

First, with the aid of descriptive statistics, research participants' demographic data were established as well as the kinds of violence experienced by each examined group. Next a qualitative analysis of the material gained from the different methods was carried out. The goal of this analysis was to obtain answers for the main research questions. The investigative process was conducted separately with each person, recorded on audiocassette, and transcripts were prepared. The material obtained was analyzed (content material was processed by using quotations from the examined person) and then interpreted psychologically.

Analysis

The resultant material was subjected to qualitative hermeneutical psychological analysis, whereby each interview was analyzed separately (Widera-Wysoczańska, 2000).

During the mother's behavior analysis, indicators from four dimensions described above were taken into consideration, some more important contents emerging from the tests were added, and for each person contents concerning the mother's relationship with the partner were sought. Categories and request models were not predetermined; they emerged from the data themselves. Answers for the questionnaire statements in "Retrospective Perception of Parental Attitudes" (RPPA) were classified according to the dimensions they belonged in. The following indicators then completed the mother's behavior analysis: "Family Childhood Abuse Questionnaire" and "Intimate Relationships".

The analysis started from repeated open-minded reading of the transcript in order to gain more sensitive view of phenomena. Next key words or sentences were discovered that appeared to be essential for an understanding of studied phenomenon. Search for words describing mother's behavior was based on the mentioned dimensions. Looking for units of meaning, i.e. fragments corresponding to the research questions was the next step. Then units relating to one issue and consisting of the same idea were put together, creating "poles of meaning", which describe different aspects of the connection of mother's behavior with the chosen partner The next step was the formation of a "personal model" of the connection of mother's behavior with the chosen partner Looking through all the graphs, I searched for important topics that I used to bring order to the interpretation of the experience, as well unnecessary information were excluded. The dominant topics referred to the type of abuses and specific and non - specific parenting features of the mothers in the childhood of studied women; features of the partner in adult life; features of the woman as a partner; features of the partner's relationship. After finishing the analysis on idiographic level research material was presented on the group level.

With the aid of cross-portrait analysis, two models connecting the mother's behavior with her chosen partner were created on a more general level. They contain types and categories based on all the cases (Tesch, 1990; Widera-Wysoczańska, 2000). One model (a type or category) was formed by combining several cases. More than three people were included in each type or category, which strengthens confidence in the trustworthiness of the types and categories in Koehn's (2007) study . In determining the level of specificity-generality of the types and categorization scheme, preference was given to a formulation that would maximize both richness and distinctiveness of the types. Previous process of analysis was done with help of quotations drawn from all the texts. This material was then the subject of the psychological interpretation in more general level, generalized for each studied group.

I adhered to the rules of validation of qualitative studies. In accordance with the triangulation criteria, I employed more than one method of collecting data. When using the criterion of persuasiveness, quotes from transcriptions allowed me to prove that interpretation is a trustworthy approach. To assess the reliability of the types and categories belonging to the model, contents assigned by the researcher to the types and categories were replicated by three competent judges, who worked independently. Each judge repeated the described procedure, assigned each unit of content to its polar meaning, and next created a personal model and a model on a more general level. A 90% accordance of assigned units of content with the generalized models, types and categories allowed that the assignment of given units of content to the certain types and categories was taken as valid. The percentage of agreement between judges and the researcher met Andersson and Nilsson's criteria (1964).

Results

First, statistics concerning violence experienced by the women under study will be presented. Then a preliminary suggestion of two parenting models, which characterize the mothers' behavior in their childhood, will be detailed . They will be described in the context of the violence which took place in their families. Presentation of the women's mates will then be the next step.

Types of abuse

These women experienced intra-familial emotional (100% of the study group), physical (60 women, 68%), and sexual (64 women, 73%) abuse. In 58 (65%) cases the father was an alcoholic and in 28 cases (32%) the mother. The persons experienced complex trauma.

Table 5-2. Traumatic events experienced by the study group of women

<table>
<tr><th colspan="4">Type of abuse</th><th>N</th><th>%</th></tr>
<tr><td colspan="4">Emotional abuse</td><td>88</td><td>100</td></tr>
<tr><td colspan="4">Physical abuse</td><td>60</td><td>68.1</td></tr>
<tr><td colspan="4">Alcoholic father</td><td>58</td><td>65.9</td></tr>
<tr><td colspan="4">Alcoholic mother</td><td>28</td><td>31.8</td></tr>
<tr><td rowspan="3">Sexual abuse</td><td>N
64</td><td>%
72.7</td><td>Emotional</td><td>58</td><td>65.9</td></tr>
<tr><td></td><td></td><td>w/o touching</td><td>38</td><td>43.1</td></tr>
<tr><td></td><td></td><td>w/ touching</td><td>42</td><td>47.7</td></tr>
</table>

These women experienced intra-familial emotional (100% of the study group), physical (60 women, 68%), and sexual (64 women, 73%) abuse. In 58 (65%) cases the father was an alcoholic and in 28 cases (32%) the mother. The persons experienced complex trauma. A distinct majority of the women experienced abuse from early childhood ("since I can remember") to when they left home, at approximately 20 years of age.

Models connecting the mothers' behavior with child and the chosen partner in adult life

Hermeneutical analysis-models were created based on the connection between the mothers' behavior in childhood and their selected mates in adult life.

The main elements of the models are phenomena relating to the context of maternal behavior (kinds of interpersonal violence taking place in the family of origin, characteristics of mother-daughter attachments (specific and non-specific), and the impact-quality of this bond on mate selection in adult life (features of the partner, of the woman and of their relationships).

Type of models of mothers - daughter attachment in the context of interpersonal abuse

Now I describe models of mother-daughter attachment in the context of interpersonal chronic, complex abuse. I distinguish two attachment models. The first I call operationally the "non-protective and distant mother", and the second the "overprotective mother".

Table 5-3. Two models of mothers - daughter attachment

MODEL I: Non-protective, distant (n=59, 67%)
Type A. Explicit distant mothers (n=12)
Type B. Ambiguous distant mothers (n=20)
Type C. Distant, exposing, seducing mothers (n=27)
MODEL II: Overprotective mothers (n=29, 32,9%)
Type A. Overprotective sexually abusive mothers (n=18)
Type B. Overprotective absent mothers (n=11)

Model I: Non-protective, distant mothers

In this model three types of mothers were distinguished:

Type A: explicit, when they plainly do not show their child love (alcoholic mothers)

Type B: ambiguous, when though distant and do not provide protection they say they love their child (sober mothers)

Type C: when though distant they seduce the child, telling it about problems with intimate life with the partner, i.e. the child's father, and at the same time believe the child should deal with him (sober mothers)

These types of mother-daughter attachment models appeared in specific contexts. In all cases the same types of abuse occurred in the family. The women experienced emotional and physical abuse. Type A mothers were alcoholics and employed different types of sexual abuse of the child (without touching, and emotional), while types B and C were not alcoholic and many of them committed emotional sexual abuse. The perpetrator of sexual abuse with touching, fondling, and penetration of intimate places was in some cases the child's father and other person.

Table 5-4. Type of chronic complex trauma as a context for distant model

Type of chronic complex trauma	
Emotional abuse Physical abuse Sexual abuse Alcoholism Perpetrators: father and/or mother and others	
A. specific abuse	B and C. specific abuse
- Alcoholism of mother and/or father - Mother a perpetrator of sexual abuse without touching: contacts with many partners in front of the child; exposing the child to sexual abuse by other persons - Father a perpetrator of sexual abuse with touching (penetration) - Did not protect their children from other perpetrators	- Alcoholism of father - Sober mother - Mother a perpetrator of emotional sexual abuse: vulgar name-calling, burdening the child to be the mother's partner - Father a perpetrator of sexual abuse: with touching (penetration), emotional and without touching - Lack of the mother's protection

These mothers had common features in their behavior. They took care of their children's food and clothing (except for the type A alcoholic mothers): “Mom provided food and clothing. The meals were always prepared but not much beside it”. They were emotionally distant, most of these mothers applied physical and sexual abuse, did not protect their children from other perpetrators, did not recognize or meet the child's needs, and had demands inappropriate to the child's age. In each model, individual, specific features appeared.

Type A. The non-protective, explicit distant mother

These mothers were emotionally distant and physically absent in the child's life, did not have time for the child, because of the drinking and constant tiredness/fatigue They did not show feelings, did not give the child warmth: "My mother never hugged me", “My mother didn't look after me much, she never took me on her lap, never said she loved me”. The child felt rejected. The child experienced shame because of the mother's drinking. The mothers also presented a physical threat: they slapped their daughters and employed sexual abuse, calling their daughters vulgar names “When she was angry with me she used to call me very vulgar names” and exposing the daughter to sexual contact with her drunk, casual partners (e.g. organizing alcoholic gatherings at home). They did not protect them from other perpetrators (the father or his drunk friends). They neither recognized nor met their child's needs. They demanded that the child carry out the parent's role by doing laundry, cooking, and cleaning. The mother was authoritative and despotic: “She used to give me orders shouting when she wanted something from me I was not allowed to discuss”; also inappropriately aggressive, she would shout at the daughter or hit her for no reason clear to the child: “When I was a child she used to beat me for anything, I usually didn’t know for what but had to apologize for that.” “She was very temperamental, she shouted and I never knew why” “There was no way of satisfying her. She believed that everything must be earned, never said that she loved me.” A similar model of a mother’s behavior was called by Heilbrun, Orr and Harrell (1966) “low control-low nurturant”, which they considered as ignoring.

Type B. The non-protective, ambiguous, distant mother

This type of mother differs from type A in her ambiguousness. These mothers are distant from their children, did not protect their daughters from emotional and physical abuse, and did not react to the child's disclosure (indirect sexual violence) of the father's sexual abuse of her. However, at the same time they said they loved their daughter: "She told me she loved me, but I had to deserve her love". These mothers demanded from their daughter’s emotional care, unconditional respect, apologies in situations where the daughter was not to blame. They were inappropriately aggressive: "By screaming or hitting me she worked off her bad mood".

Type C. The distant, exposing, seducing mother

These mothers left their children emotionally: "She was absent in my life.", and similar to type A and B mothers, they were emotionally distant: "She didn't show me warm feelings, she was cold, didn't take care of me". The mother showed her helplessness in life: "She was always tired, busy, and couldn't cope with anything" and separated herself from the daughter and demanded that the daughter not disturb her. They did not protect their daughters from sexual abuse (indirect sexual violence) and denied its existence: "She pretended that everything was OK" even when the child disclosed that the father touched her in intimate places. They used their children to satisfy their own needs, telling them about unsuccessful intimate situations with their partner, most often the child's father, used the child in conflicts with the father and demanded from the daughter that she tend to him: "Mother ordered me to sleep in one room with my constantly drunk father so I could take care of him when he came home drunk or woke up in the night and needed something. Mother had her own room".,

The authoritative mother demanded from the daughter absolute obedience: "That was the only way I could get a little bit of acceptance".

Table 5-5. Behaviors of the distant mothers in the childhood of the studied women

Common features		
Basic care Emotional distance Physical violence threat Lack of protection Not meeting the child's needs Demands inappropriate to the child's age Inappropriately aggressive reactions		
Specific features		
A. Distant, explicit non-protective mother	B. distant, ambiguous mother	C. distant, exposing, seducing mother
-Neglect of basic care -Plainly does not show affection to the child, is cold - threatens emotionally: emotional abandonment, rejection, emotional absence in the child's life shaming the child (drinking) -Threatens physically: beatings, lack of protection, emotional violence, indirect sexual violence (exposure to sexual contacts with others) - Demands unsuitable for the child's age -Imposing the role of parent and parent caregiver on the child (washing, cooking, cleaning) -Authoritarian, despotic/domineering - Alcoholic	- Emotional threat, emotional distance + love declared only verbally + inappropriate demands, accusing the child, blaming - Physical threat, beatings, no protection, no reaction to disclosure of sexual abuse - Role: burdening the child with emotional care of the mother (coping with her emotions) -Despotic, demanding, demanding absolute respect - Sober	-Emotional threat, distance, abandonment -Physical threat, denial of sexual violence, no protection, no reaction to disclosure of abuse - Roles and boundaries : using the child to satisfy their own needs, forced to listen to intimate confessions about the bad partner using the daughter in conflicts with the father - Mother's helplessness, Demanding absolute respect and obedience - Sober

Model II: Overprotective mothers

In both cases (A and B) emotional and sexual harassment occurred in the family. In type A some of the father were alcoholic and mother had problems with alcohol. In case of part of studied women their mothers were perpetrators of sexual abuse; the women did not report physical abuse. In type B the mother left the daughter and sexual abuse in some cases occurred, the perpetrator of which was not a person from the nearest family

Table 5-6. Type of chronic complex interpersonal trauma as a context for overprotective mothers

Type of trauma	
Emotional abuse Sexual abuse Perpetrators: father and/or mother and grandfather	
Specific abuse	
A. sexually abusive mothers	B. absent mothers
Father alcoholic Mother with at least alcohol problem Father and mother perpetrators of sexual abuse with/ without touching (penetration)	Physical abandonment of the child by the mother Sexual abuse (e.g. grandfather)

Material shows two types of overprotective mother. All of them tended to the child's food and clothing. Their behavior shows high, intrusive control. They created a symbiotic relationship with the daughter. They did not protect their daughters from sexual abuse by the father and other persons (e.g. partners of the drunk mother),if it took place/occurred. They applied pathological control over the child, making the child dependent on them and their "love" and simultaneously transgressing the child's emotional and physical boundaries, using the child to satisfy their own needs, demanding to be cared for. They demanded absolute obedience. They did not recognize or satisfy the child's real needs. This type of mother behavior could spoils a child by making him or her exceptionally demanding and incapable in later life doing without love.

Type A are mothers who, besides the father, sexually abused their daughters and did not protect their daughters from sexual abuse by the father (touching, penetration, pornography). Type B mothers abandoned their daughters, going to another city or country or leaving the child for the grandparents to bring up. Sexual abuse also occurred here for a few women, with the perpetrator being the grandfather or a person from outside the family.

Type A Overprotective sexually abusive mothers

Overprotective mothers who committed sexual abuse (most of them had problems with alcohol) created symbiotic relationships with their daughters. They pathologically and intrusively controlled their daughters, not allowing them to develop their autonomy and independence: “She always knew what was good for me and what I wanted. She forced me to satisfy these imaginary needs invented by her. She had no idea about my real needs.” They are childish. They sexually abused their daughters: They touched the child’s intimate places - calling it child care (washing an adolescent child’s intimate places), exposed themselves before the child (walking naked), masturbated in the child's presence, had sex (caresses, intercourse) with different partners in front of the child: “She used to trespass my boundaries, she used to touch me in very unexpected moments, she used to talk about my breasts in front of men.” Simultaneously they did not protect them from the father when it was necessary. They demanded emotional care and attention from the daughter: "My mother overwhelmed me with her expectations." They accused the daughter of lack of interest in relations with the mother: "Mother always told me that I didn't love her, especially when I didn't want her to touch me in a way that embarrassed me, or that I didn’t want to sleep with her." In this way the mothers aroused feelings of guilt and shame, demonstrating that they were deeply hurt by the child: “Her suffering expression never failed to produce a feeling of guilt in me. I had to approach her.” At the same time they saw their daughters as rivals: “She used to say she was prettier than me.”

Type B Overprotective, absent mothers

These mothers were characterized by many contradictions. They abandoned their child, going to another city or country, and at the same time treated their daughter as a friend she could confide in or whom she encouraged to be open: “I was her best friend”. On the one hand they were physical distant from their daughters because of their physical absence, and on the other gave the child love, care, and warmth. They were controlling, and authoritarian, demanding absolute obedience and expecting their daughters to live according to their notions. They would leave the daughter alone, demanding that she fulfill the role of an adult partner, parent, and possibly caregiver for the father: “She used to burden me with things surpassing my age that shouldn’t be left to children, I was to pay the rent, look after my ill father when she moved to another town." A similar type of maternal pattern Heilbrun, Orr and Harrell (1966) called "high control-low nurturant," which entails "rejection".

Table 5-7. Overprotective mothers' behaviors in the childhood of the studied women

<table>
<tr><td colspan="2">Common features
OVERPROTECTIVE</td></tr>
<tr><td colspan="2">Basic care
High, intrusive, pathological control and low care
Not allowing the child to develop autonomy and independence
Seducing the child
Lack of understanding the needs, dream of child
Not meeting the child's needs
Lack of agreement
Demands inappropriate to the child's age - care of the mother
Demanding absolute obedience</td></tr>
<tr><td colspan="2">Specific features</td></tr>
<tr><td>A.
sexually abusive mothers</td><td>B.
absent mothers</td></tr>
<tr><td>-Emotional threats: they showed too many overwhelming feelings, lack of support; blamed the child for the mother's bad emotional state when the child didn't submit to enough intimacy; shamed the child; talked about the child's body in an embarrassing way; accused the daughter of lack of involvement in relations with the mother
-Physical threat: trespassing intimate (bodily) borders; lack of support
-Focus on mother's emotional and bodily needs
-Roles: the child should be the mother's partner or a plaything, always take her side, comfort her; blurred generational borders; mother demands to be looked after emotionally by her child, child must be on the mother's side, child must console the mother;
-Over-control, no child autonomy
-daughter as a rival
-Mothers at least with alcohol problem</td><td>-Physical and emotional threat: physically abandoning the child; no care, warmth
-Roles, boundaries: does not listen to demands from the child
-Controlling, authoritarian, demanding unconditional obedience, daughter must live according to her expectations and ideas, the child must be the mother's friend
-The child must assume the role of a parent
-The child must look after the father when the mother is absent</td></tr>
</table>

The mate selection in the adult life

I shall now describe the types of partner relationships which the studied women reported. They shall be shown in the context of the two mother-daughter attachment models. The quality of the current partner relationships seem to be a consequence of interpersonal trauma experienced in childhood (the types of abuse) and quality of mother-daughter attachment.

How do the studied women who had distant and overprotective mothers describe their choice of a partner? Partner relations of women brought up by distant mothers are very similar in the three types of parenting attitudes discussed before. The partners are withdrawn from domestic life, without initiative, and also cold and domineering (in types B and C). Some of them were alcoholic, aggressive, treacherous, and sexually abused their daughters (if they had any):"I was suppressed, he used emotional and physical violence against me, and I was sexually abused." "My husband was aggressive, occasionally violent, and untruthful." These women, whose needs were not fulfilled in childhood and who were burdened with caring for the mother and father (type C - the child is sacrificed for the father), are submissive and do not recognize their own needs: "She couldn't express her needs", but are focused on the needs of the domineering partner and are subordinate to him. They do not believe in their own potential and consider themselves unattractive. Sexually abused in childhood, they feel aversion to sex, but agree to intercourse out of fear of rejection: "I submit to sex for fear of offending him". They mistake mercy for love. Lack of (mutual) understanding is the relationship's main characteristic: They are not able to talk to one another and cannot understand the needs of each other.

The partner relationships of women brought up by overprotective mothers are different in types A and B. Women who were sexually abused by their father and mother and were shamed and blamed by the mother for a lack of involvement in the relationship with the mother have problems with their sexual identity and some of them enter into homosexual relationships having a mother-daughter character. Their partners (homo- or heterosexual) are controlling, accusatory, and emotionally introverted. These women were addicted to their partners' presence. "I didn't feel attractive in their company, they didn't support me, but they just had to be there, I couldn't live without such kind of love." In their relationships, these women in the study (similar to those in the last group) did not understand their own needs: "The partner's needs were a priority, even at my expense. I simply wasn't there; neither were any of my needs or dreams". Their relationships are characterized as attraction-distancing. "When the partner was involved, I retreated, and when the partner escaped, I became involved."

Table 5-8. Partner choice by distanced mothers' daughters

DISTANT MOTHERS		
A	B	C
Features of the partner Withdrawn - no involvement - no initiative - aversion to conversations Perpetrator - alcoholism - women are playthings - demands attention and care Features of the woman - over-responsible - does not understand and does not express own needs - focused on the partner's needs - fear of being abandoned Features of the relationship - no understanding - no communication	Features of the partner Withdrawn - no involvement - no initiative - aversion to conversations - cold and strict - abandoning - treacherous Perpetrator - aggressive - treacherous Features of the woman - controlling - over-protective - dependent (emotionally and financially) - submissive - does not understand and does not express own needs - no belief in own potential - aversion to sex - agreeing to sex for the partner - fear of abandonment Features of the relationship - no understanding - no communication	Features of the partner Withdrawn - no involvement - no initiative - escape - domineering Perpetrator - sexual abuse of the daughter - alcoholism Features of the woman - domineering - overprotective - dependent (emotionally and financially) - submissive - does not understand and does not express own needs - focused on the partner's needs - feels unattractive - no sexual satisfaction Features of the relationship - no understanding - no communication - mistook mercy for love

In type B, where the mothers of the studied women on the one hand abandoned their daughters and on the other felt over-responsible for them, the women had partners who were withdrawn and who lacked initiative, who treated their women as playthings. Women in these relationships are controlling and domineering, over-responsible for organization and domestic chores "In the relationship I was a domineering, over-responsible person. It's me who organized domestic life, but I couldn't show any warm feelings or say 'no' when I didn't want something." They focus on the partner's problems and needs: "Our life was subordinated to him and his needs", are emotionally dependent on the partner: "I used to give in for fear of being rejected; I didn't want to be alone as I was in my childhood." They do not recognize, understand or express their own needs. They confuse sex with love: "I was treated like someone used to satisfying man's sexual needs, I mistook sex for love, and I didn't know my boundaries." They feel fear of being rejected when they refuse or avoid sex. They seek a father in much older partners: "I used to have partners much older than me. These relationships were superficial, devoid of deeper feelings."

Table 5-9. Mate selection by overprotective mothers' daughters

OVERPROTECTIVE	
A	B
Features of the partner - controlling - accusatory - emotionally introverted Features of the woman - does not recognize and express own needs - addicted to a partner - over-responsible Features of the relationship A. Homosexual B. Heterosexual - conversations (only in homosexual relationships) - attraction-distancing	Features of the partner Withdrawn - no involvement - no initiative - abandoning Perpetrator - treats women as playthings Features of the woman - controlling and domineering - overprotective - focused on the partner's problems and needs - emotionally dependent on the partner - does not recognize and express own needs - sex: lack of boundaries, confuses sex with love, fear of rejection if she refuses sex, avoids sex, looks for a father in older partners Features of the relationship - problems in understanding

Summary comments

This research has focused on the qualities of mother and child attachment occurring in a family where the child has experienced interpersonal trauma, and on its influence in mate selection in adult life. Research has shown a tendency toward insecure attachments affecting adult relationships with partners. These insecurities in childhood - physical and emotional distance of the mother or her over-protectiveness (over-control) of the child - may lead to the eventual choice of a partner who is emotionally frigid, uninvolved in the relationship, controlling, emotionally, physically, and also sexually violent (toward both the children and the partner), who focuses on his own needs, ignores the partner's needs, and treats her like a plaything or a servant. The woman is over-responsible toward the family, does not recognize her own needs and, for fear of losing her partner, tolerates even violence to herself and her children. Sex is perceived as a compulsion; they mistake sex for love and love for mercy. They may look for older partners and some of them have homosexual relationships, and only in such are there some talks between partners. The other relationships are silent with some conflicts solving problems. Apparently parental overprotection has been regarded as similarly harmful, like deprivation of care, in its consequences, and has been blamed for having a determining influence on the development of problems in various areas of life, including the interpersonal area. It is worth considering that research results may indicate intergenerational transmission of abuse in the family.

Mothers' behavioral models presented above concentrate on their dysfunctional aspects. Such perceptions are made by daughters who had experienced interpersonal trauma in their childhood and who took part in therapy. Women from functional families surely would show a different - that is, a more positive - picture of their guardians and mate selections.

Our understanding of this issue is enriched because we are listening to the perspectives of clients themselves. However, the completed research provides grounds for generating additional hypotheses and can be considered as an introduction to further studies of the influence of the mother's attachment phenomenon on mate selection.

It is also known that a woman's good-quality relationship with her partner is also influenced by the quality of the father-daughter bond. Therefore research should be continued to study the influence of father-figure relationships on both women's and men's choices of a partner and the influence of the mother-son relationship on mate selection by men. Let us remember that although women do choose partners, these partners have also chosen women with certain characteristics; so not only the women's past but also the men's past lead to their encounter. Being analyzed additionally is material concerning changes in a relationship with the mother caused by participation in therapy and the impact of these changes on mate selection and the relationship with him. At this time, such obtained material is being studied. I hope it will improve our awareness of parental influence on our adult life and on building close relationships.

So that changes in partner relationships are lasting, it is necessary that persons who experienced chronic trauma go through the entire therapeutic process. The lessons of attachment learned during couple-therapy help people heal adult relationships.

PART III

THE DEVELOPMENT OF PERSONALITY DISORDERS

CHAPTER SIX

TRAUMATIC AND NON-TRAUMATIC PATHS OF BORDERLINE PERSONALITY DISORDER DEVELOPMENT

LIDIA CIERPIAŁKOWSKA

Introduction

The paper is focused on the problem of relationships between mental disorders, especially borderline personality disorders, and trauma. An observation made by clinicians and psychotherapists suggesting that traumatic experiences in childhood and adolescence significantly increase the risk of mental disorders has been verified in a quite substantial number of currently available studies that compared patients with different mental disorders. Although practical observations have often been confirmed, little is known yet about the impact of trauma on the development of psychological path mechanisms underpinning specific clinical syndromes. As was the case with PTSD, the focus of research interest in the field of personality disorders is mainly on explaining the role and consequences of trauma in the development of a pathological personality structure or organization. Since the conception by O. Kernberg (1976, 1996) deals with the influence of early childhood trauma on intrapsychic mechanisms and on maintenance of specific levels pathology in personality organization, the presentation of theoretical assumptions and conclusions drawn from their empirical verifications have received major attention in this paper.

Around the concept of trauma

Over a century ago Josef Breuer & Sigmund Freud (1892/2001) published their study *On the Psychic Mechanisms of Hysterical Phenomena*, where interesting views on psychological and neurological effects of trauma experienced in early childhood by their female patients can be found. The authors state that "…in the case of "traumatic" hysteria it is trauma that is the cause of the symptom" (*ibid.*, p. 11) which "… disappears immediately and irretrievably if a quite clear memory of the event that had elicited it could be awakened" (*ibid.*, p. 13). A few years later in *A General Introduction to Psychoanalysis* Freud (1916-1917/2000, p. 260) defined trauma as

> …an experience that within a short time brings into spiritual life so strong an increase in stimuli that the individual can neither get rid of them nor processes them in a normal way, which must result in constant disturbances in his/her energy system.

In psychoanalysis trauma is defined as a kind of psychic experience evoking a shock that prevents the individual's adequate response, which results in a long-term pathogenic influence of the experience on the developing psychic organization (Laplanche and Pontalis 1992).

Besides paradigmatic approaches, in the study of trauma an important role is assigned to integrative approaches often originating from regulatory theories of personality and behavior. In these theories trauma is usually defined as a unique single event or a long-term effect of external circumstances involving either a direct risk to the individual's life or health, or a very significant reduction in ability to assimilate the experience, which leads to a destabilization or disintegration of the existing personality organization (Pearlman and Saakvitne, 1995; Terr, 1991; Martens, 2005). Objective, external events are clearly distinguished from a subjectively experienced stress load, which depending on the individual's characteristics may be variously appraised and emotionally responded to. Among various subjective factors differentiating the individual's appraisal of a stress load, particular attention has been paid to temperamental traits and the level of received social support (cf. Lis-Turlejska, 1998, 2002; Korkeila, Lehtinen, Bijl et al., 2003).

Since so many events in human life meet the criteria of traumaticity, considerable attention has been devoted to defining major criteria that would enable a valid classification of such events (for a review see Dudek, 2003; Garland, 2009). A developmental perspective helps to explain the role of trauma in the origin of mental disorders, since in this framework two pivotal questions are taken into account: (1) the life stage in which a stress overload was experienced - childhood, adolescence, or adulthood, and (2) the character of stress - and more precisely, whether it was repetitive or associated with a single event. On the grounds of the first criterion, i.e. the life stage of the stressful experience occurrence, childhood trauma was distinguished from adulthood trauma. The former is considered to be more important than the latter in the development of mental disorders other than post-traumatic stress disorder (PTSD). Childhood trauma is frequently termed "relational" in contradistinction to other traumatic experiences such as accidents or disasters. The second criterion allows for the classification of the trauma into two categories: acute or long-term (chronic). Terr (1991) distinguished two types of trauma: type I includes difficult incidental events, while type II denotes repeated traumatic experiences frequently associated with stressful family relationships and behaviors of parents or siblings (e.g. neglect, sexual abuse, violence). More recently Allen and Lauterbach (2007) distinguished a type III trauma, involving a mixture of type I and type II traumatic experiences, and probably leading to the most severe mental disorders. Even though some research findings suggest that chronic trauma experienced in childhood results in internalization of problems (e.g. anxiety disorders, depression), while incidental trauma tends to produce rather externalization (behavior disorders, antisocial personality disorder) (Kiser, Heston, Millsap & Pruitt, 1991; Martens, 2005), the results of more recent studies (cf. Allen and Lauterbach, 2007; Weber, Rockstroh, Bergelt et al., 2008) are not so unambiguous.

Trauma and paths of mental disorders development

Recent research findings concerning the relationship of adverse and traumatic experiences in childhood, adolescence, and adulthood to the onset of mental disorders, show that an above-normal stress load in childhood is related to various mental health problems, including depressive disorders (Heim, Plotsky & Nemeroff 2004), schizophrenia (Read, VanOs, Morrison et al., 2005), anxiety disorders with posttraumatic stress disorder (PTSD) (Scheller-Gilkey, Moynes, Cooper et al., 2004), personality disorders (Martens 2005), or substance dependence (Dragon 2008).

Results of successive studies prompted researchers to ask a question about relationships between the time of trauma onset and vulnerability to mental disorders. In research projects currently under way attempts are made to describe and explain: 1) what are the implications of relational trauma and trauma due to critical life events for health and mental disorders, and 2) what specific intrapsychic path mechanisms develop depending on the stage of psychic structure development at which trauma has occurred. The relationships between the traumatic stress impact and other factors increasing vulnerability to mental disorders, particularly temperamental characteristics, are in the focus of interest of many Polish clinicians and researchers (Strelau et al., 2004; Dragon 2008).

At present three different paths are distinguished of mental disorders development in consequence of stress overload at various stages of human life. Each of the paths is assumed to reflect a specific mechanism underpinning the development of psychopathology. The paths are illustrated in Fig. 6-1.

Figure 6-1. Trauma and paths of mental disorders development

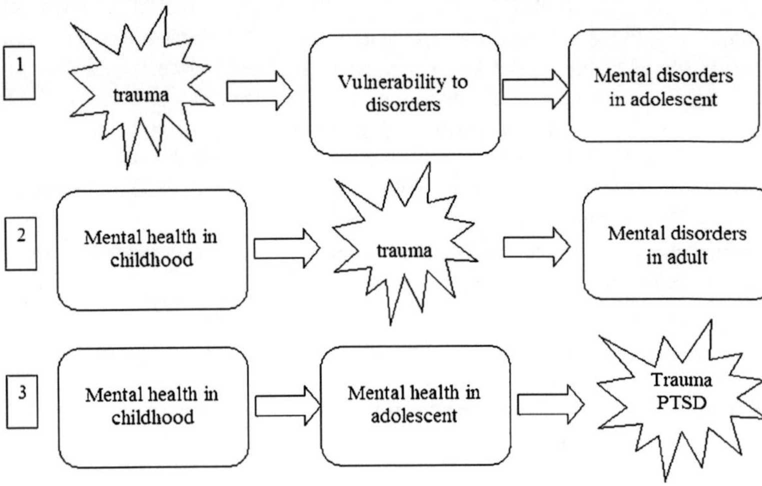

Path 1 shows the relationships between stressful experiences (stress load) in early childhood and an enhanced tendency to either externalization or internalization of problems in adolescence, increasing the risk of various mental disorders in adulthood. High stress levels may affect functional and structural systems (including the neuroendocrine system) that are developing during this period in the brain. The resulting abnormalities are most often manifested as an increased reactivity to various stimuli and events, activating strong affective responses. If such responses are maintained over long periods of time, a chronic state of increased excitation ensues in the individual.

Early childhood relational trauma is in the focus of interest of psychoanalysts who have posed a few hypotheses concerning its effect on the child's personality formation. Generally, it is assumed in the object relations theory that relational trauma may lead to the defense mechanism of splitting which determines the level of pathology in personality organization (Kernberg 1996; Holmes, Brown, Mansell et al., 2005), or is reflected in the inner working model of attachment developing at that time and determining patterns of the individual's cognitive-emotional behaviors towards self and others (Bowlby, 2008; Blatt, Auerbach & Levy, 1997).

Path 2 shows that the course of development until adolescence has been probably optimal, but after a traumatic event a breakdown of the hitherto utilized coping strategies ensues and the individual's school achievements no longer are for him/her a source of satisfaction. As mentioned before, the impact of trauma at that time results in activation of the paths of either the internalization or externalization of problems and difficulties, leading to the onset of different mental disorders. While externalization of problems in adulthood frequently leads to behavior disorders, substance dependence or antisocial personality disorders, internalization is highly correlated with depression, anxiety disorders or dependent personality disorder. Vulnerability to various mental disorders is significantly enhanced by school failure (Masten, Rossman & Long, 2005).

Finally, path 3 illustrates the sources and mechanism of the onset of either acute or posttraumatic stress disorders (ASD and PTSD, respectively) in a person whose psychological development has followed a relatively normal course until adulthood. A review of studies on PTSD prevalence allows one to conclude that: 1) it is the most often diagnosed mental disorder (PTSD lifetime prevalence rate is about 8-9% of the general population; cf. Hidalgo and Davidson, 2000); 2) a majority of people who have experienced a traumatic event manifest no PTSD symptoms (Lis-Turlejska 1998); 3) most people diagnosed with PTSD experience spontaneous remission, recover and are symptom-free (Rothbaum and Foa, 1992). Among many sociodemographic predictors of PTSD onset the most often reported factors include gender (even though men more frequently experience traumatic events, it is women who display more PTSD symptoms), age and place of residence (more extensive symptoms are seen more often in young residents of large urban agglomerations), and health status (people with mental disorders more often suffer from PTSD than the mentally sane) (Dragon, 2008).

Relationships between experiencing a traumatic event and PTSD are to a large extent modified by biological and psychological factors that may either serve a protective function or increase the risk for the disorder onset. Not only specific temperamental characteristics, especially severe neuroticism and introversion, are crucial for an increased risk of PTSD (Strelau et al., 2004), but also some personality traits (with a tendency to activate the mechanism of dissociation being the center of researchers' attention) (Spitzer, Barnow, Freyberger & Grabe, 2006; Löffler-Stastka, Szerencsics & Blüml , 2009). In the trauma literature the notion of dissociation is used in three different meanings referring to diverse conceptions of the phenomenon. Dissociation is construed, firstly, as a lack of integration of positive and negative self- and object-representations in the personality organization; secondly, as alternative (two or more) states of consciousness; and thirdly, as a defense mechanism that can be either developmental or pathologic (cf. Holmes et al., 2006).

Numerous attempts have been made to verify empirically the above-described models of the effect of trauma on mental disorders development. Particularly noteworthy seems to be the recent comparative study conducted by Katja Weber and her co-workers (2008). Participants in the study were 96 inpatients of a Center for Psychiatry and 31 volunteers without mental disorders. The main aim of the research was to find out whether stressful experiences during childhood, adolescence and adulthood are related to different mental disorders including schizophrenia, depression, substance dependence, and personality disorders. It was hypothesized that: a) stress load would be higher in patients with mental disorders than in subjects from the comparative group; b) severity of mental disorders should be related to the number of traumatic events and to experiencing stress at an earlier stage of life; c) the nature of mutual relations between adverse experiences and psychopathology would be similar to that described for traumatic events and PTSD symptoms or delusions.

Inter- and intragroup comparisons included the number of stressful events and the amount of stress load during childhood (under the age of 6), adolescence, and adulthood (using the *Early Trauma Inventory* to measure general trauma, physical punishment neglect and sexual abuse), as well as PTSD severity (assessed using the *Posttraumatic Stress Diagnostic Scale*). Severity of the participants' mental disorders was assessed using three instruments measuring the level of their general functioning in various areas of life, as well as severity of symptomatology of depression and other forms of psychopathology.

A majority of the hypotheses posed were confirmed. Both the number of stressful events and the amount of stress load turned out to be higher in patients with mental disorders than in subjects from the comparative group. Moreover, the patients as compared to subjects without mental disorders more often experienced family violence, as well as an at least 3-month separation from the biological mother during preadolescence (before puberty). They had also lower school achievements. Intragroup comparisons indicated that among all the subgroups of patients those with personality disorders had the highest number of adverse events and trauma load levels not only in their prenatal life, but also in their early childhood and pre-pubertal period. Higher stress levels were noted in patients with depression than in those who were substance dependent or suffering from schizophrenia. When the patients were divided into subgroups by the stress load experienced during different periods of life, the "high stress" group turned out to consist mostly of patients with depression or personality disorders and the "low stress" with substance dependence, while that of "moderate stress" included, above all, patients with schizophrenia (Weber, Rockstroh, Borgelt et al., 2008).

The findings corroborate the assumption about a sensitive developmental period when an interaction of genetic predispositions (prenatal stress) with traumatic stress load leads to the development of mental disorders, first and foremost to personality and mood disorders. No confirmation was found for any direct relationships between stress load and severity of mental disorders in PTSD cases. Among different personality disorders particular attention is paid to borderline personality disorder, rather commonly regarded in the literature as psychopathology due to childhood trauma (cf. Watson, Chiton, Fairchild & Whewell, 2006; Löffler-Stastka, Szerencsics & Blüml , 2009).

Paths of borderline personality disorder development

According to psychoanalytic, cognitive and cognitive-behavioral theories, personality disorders develop across lifespans from childhood through adolescence to adulthood. Although in each of the approaches different intrapsychic mechanisms underpinning the development of such disorders are described, nevertheless similar assumptions are made regarding the etiological role of biological and environmental factors (Kernberg 1980, 1996; Pretzer and Beck, 1996; Linehan 1987, 2007).

Generally, taking into account the proportions of temperamental and familial determinants, clinicians describe two paths of the borderline personality disorder development: traumatic and non-traumatic. In the non-traumatic path a major role is ascribed to various characteristics of the central nervous system reflected in temperamental traits that predispose the individual to very violent, long-lasting, negative emotional responses to relatively weak external stimuli (Graybar and Boutilier, 2002; Magnavita, 2004). Traumatic events, familial or non-familial, are believed to play a less important role. The opposite holds true for the other mechanism considered to result, above all, from the individual's experiencing a considerable stress load in early childhood due to emotional neglect, abandonment, and physical, mental, or sexual abuse (Linehan, 1987; Kernberg, 1996; Graybar and Boutilier, 2002).

In contemporary psychoanalysis, especially in the object relations theory, attempts are made to explain the effect of trauma on the development and functioning of the psychic apparatus in terms of dissociation defined either as a defense mechanism or as a specific psychological process leading to a pathological personality structure or organization. The term *dissociation* considered as a defense mechanism is used interchangeably with *splitting*.

As early as the mid-1900s Glover (1943, cf. Thoma and Kachele, 1996) postulated that primary emotional experiences of early childhood constitute ego-nuclei that owing to the synthesizing function of the psyche become integrated into a relatively consistent ego structure. In consequence of strong negative experiences (trauma) this structure may disintegrate into primary ego nuclei at different stages of the individual's life. A pathological dissociation process that makes the attainment of normal integration impossible was described by Bion (1996), when explaining the consequences of the mother's difficulty in containing negative feelings of her child. If the mother lacks the capability of understanding, containing and neutralizing the child's negative affects, the process of "marking" his/her inner experiences becomes disturbed, and deficits in this respect not only lead to an exacerbation of affective disregulation, but also impede the normal development of self- and object representations. Disturbances of the mentalization process related to the child's experiencing extremely negative affective states in the relationship with the mother were pointed out by Fonagy and co-workers (2002). When discussing consequences of stressful experiences, with emotional neglect during early childhood first and foremost, the authors emphasized the role of internalization of negative self-object-affect relationships leading to an impediment of psychological development and dissociation proneness. However, it seems that the most significant contribution to the understanding of the effect of trauma on the development of pathology in borderline personality organization was that by O. Kernberg.

In the psychological structure development and formation model proposed by Kernberg (1976), a pivotal role is assigned to internalization in the form of introjection, identification, and ego-self identity in object relations. In the development of this structure five stages are distinguished. In stage I of normal autism the child does not differentiate between self and the environment and experiences only either a decrease or increase of tension resulting from either gratification or non-fulfillment of his/her needs. At that time memory traces are formed of positive, gratifying experiences, as well as of negative, frustrating relations with the mother that underpin the primary undifferentiated self-object representations. In stage II - of normal symbiosis - a primarily undifferentiated constellation of self-object-affect units is formed around positive gratifying, and negative frustrating relations with the mother. Since the child's psychic apparatus is incapable of integrating mutually opposite affective values, a distinction has to be made between libidinal and aggressive representations using the mechanism of splitting, which serves a positive role at this developmental stage. Next, in stage III - of distinction between self-representations and object-representations - a process begins of differentiating self-object representations into *good* self and *good* object, followed by differentiation within the negative representations, into *bad* self and *bad* object. Towards the end of this stage, splitting serves an increasingly less important function, being replaced by repression and other more mature defense mechanisms. If the course of this process is abnormal due to biological or environmental (trauma) factors in the child's life increasing his/her aggression, the development of personality organization becomes fixed. Stages IV and V are periods of self- and object integration, as well as of the development of higher-level psychological structures, i.e. the ego and the superego. At that time *good* and *bad* self-representations become consolidated into the so-called self-system, almost simultaneously with consolidation of *good* and *bad* object representations into holistic object representations. Moreover, there is an increasing integration within the psychological structures of the ego and the superego, including various experiences of the child related to his/her maturation in the sphere of dependence, autonomy, and identification (Kernberg, 1976).

According to Kernberg (1976, 1996), borderline personality organization is determined by an intrapsychic conflict and fixation of the individual's development in stage III, i.e. in the period of differentiation between self-representations and object-representations. The conflict between libido and aggression drives is enhanced at this stage due to two reasons: firstly, because of a constitutional factor resulting in higher aggression levels in these children, and secondly, due to their negative traumatic experiences in the relationship with the mother. Both these factors increase the level of negative affects, especially aggression, which leads to an enhancement of the splitting mechanism. The latter enables the child to maintain a real relationship with his/her mother and project negative experiences onto other objects in the environment.

At this stage of object-relations formation the defense mechanism of splitting is a developmentally desirable phenomenon, the more so that in the next stage of integration of positive and negative aspects of both self-representations and object-representations it is replaced by a more mature mechanism of repression. However, if a conflict between libido and aggression drives arising under such circumstances becomes additionally enhanced by the child's constitutionally determined higher aggression level and/or by traumatic experiences resulting from a lack of appropriate response of the object to his/her needs for bonding, then splitting becomes more pronounced. Exacerbation of conflict and of conflict-related anxiety results in an increased tendency to separate libidinally invested self- and object representations from their aggressively invested counterparts, even though the process of their differentiation has not finished yet. According to Kernberg (1976, p. 146), both the described course of differentiation between self and object and its intrapsychic consequences are characteristic of borderline personality organization.

Kernberg (2004) described three structurally different types of pathological personality organization determined by diverse defense mechanisms: psychotic personality organization determined by primitive dissociation; borderline organization with the underlying mechanism of splitting, and neurotic organization determined by repression. While psychotic organization, the most unstable and undifferentiated of the three, results from fixation of the self-object-affect representations in stages I or II, the most consolidated neurotic organization is formed as a result of attaining the final stage of development, i.e. stage IV, of a preliminary integration of self-and object-representations and emergence of the ego and the superego. Borderline personality organization is an outcome of the development stopping at the stage of an unfinished differentiation process and of the predomination of splitting over repression. Kernberg considers this type of organization to be characteristic of a vast majority of personality disorders distinguished in the DSM-IV.

Particular levels of pathology in borderline personality organization reflect and show evidence of a fixation in the psychic apparatus development that can be seen in the following areas: 1) internalized self-object relations and associated affects; 2) defensive operations of the ego and the superego structures (layers); and 3) stability of self (identity) and object. Depending on the severity of disorders, all the pathologies of character can be arranged along a continuum from the least to most severe.

As it has been noted earlier, Kernberg (2004) relates the phenomenon of dissociation to the action of primary defense mechanisms, particularly of splitting, projection, and projective identification that predominate in both borderline and psychotic personality organization. These mechanisms support the individual's proneness either to primary idealization associated with a sense of omnipotence, or to devaluation with feelings of absolute worthlessness and dependence. This level of character organization is present in most patients with cluster A and cluster B personality disorders diagnosed by the DSM-IV-TR (2000) criteria, i.e. in those with schizotypal, cyclothymic, histrionic, narcissistic, sadomasochistic, borderline, paranoid, or antisocial personalities. Particular types of personality disorders belonging to the pathology of borderline personality organization differ from each other in two main dimensions, namely the level of introversion-extraversion and aggressiveness.

Among various attempts at empirical verification of O. Kernberg's conception of the role of dissociation resulting from early childhood trauma in the formation of borderline personality organization pathology, the study conducted by Vienna psychoanalysts H. Löffler-Stastka, M. Szerencsics and V. Blüml (2009) seems particularly noteworthy. Their subjects were 52 patients aged 20-66 years, diagnosed with borderline personality organization by experienced psychiatrists using the Kernberg structured interview. All the subjects were hospitalized because of the necessity for crisis intervention, had no criminal record, and their participation in the study was voluntary. A number of instruments were used to measure dissociative symptoms severity, the amount of childhood trauma, personality pathology (*Shedler-Westen Assessment Procedure-200*, SWAP, and *Personality Pathology Q-sort*, SWAP.QT), as well as affective experiences (intensity, lability and negative affectivity proneness), and affective regulation (with three dimensions: reality orientation, externalization, and avoidance proneness). All the subjects displayed symptoms of at least one type of personality disorder by the DSM-IV criteria, and some of them had also other Axis I disorders including mood or anxiety disorders, disorders related to substance abuse, and psychoses. As regards experienced trauma, the subjects scored higher on the scales of emotional neglect, physical and mental violence, while scoring lower on the scales of physical neglect, sexual abuse, experiencing inconsistency, and belittling/repression.

Assumptions and hypotheses of the study were confirmed to a limited extent by the findings. Statistically significant relationships were found between dissociative symptoms severity on some scales (of amnesia, preoccupation, derealization and conversion) and trauma load resulting from such experiences during childhood as inconsistency, mental violence, and sexual abuse. Experiences related to emotional violence turned out to be correlated most strongly with the general dissociation level, which corresponds to the results reported in other studies investigating patients with borderline personality organization. Intimidation, affective abuse, intrusive style of controlling children is the causes of significant dissociations within self and objects, and such dissociations may be activated during adulthood under various circumstances.

The obtained results show negative correlations between dissociative symptoms severity and hostile externalizing-dysphoric personality. In this category of patients hard-to-bear negative affects such as fury or hatred are not externalized, but dissociated. This would mean that "successful" dissociation of negative affects makes hostile-externalizing behaviors unnecessary. According to Kernberg (2004), dissociative symptoms can be interpreted as the individual's efforts to escape from objects full of hatred and aggression into a dissociated world full of ideal and omnipotent objects. Dissociative symptoms seem to be complex ways of repressing hatred owing to the previous mechanism of splitting.

From the methodological perspective the study has some flaws, among which the major one is that most of the research instruments were self-report scales. Moreover, much to the authors' surprise, such tools as the SWAP and SWAP-QT used for the measurement of personality dimensions were probably not diagnostic for the study sample. Nevertheless, valuable data were collected corroborating complex relationships between dissociation severity and trauma load during early childhood in the group of patients with various types of personality disorders considered as borderline personality organization according to Kernberg.

Final remarks

Theoretical conceptions and the resulting research models strive to explain relationships between experiencing trauma at various stages of life and the development of Axis I and II mental disorders (DSM-IV-TR, 2000, 2008). Almost all studies confirm that trauma experienced during childhood and adolescence increases vulnerability to various mental health problems, while traumatic experiences in adulthood increase the likelihood of PTSD onset. Among various events the most detrimental turned out to be neglect and emotional violence.

There may be different paths of personality disorders development, depending on the level of biological and environmental risks in the individual's life. Vulnerability to this type of mental disorder is increased not only by trauma, but also by a specific configuration of temperamental traits. In psychoanalysis attempts are made to explain the path mechanism underpinning the development of borderline personality organization due to trauma in early childhood. Particular attention is paid to the dissociation process differentially affecting personality organization formed at successive stages of life. At present major research efforts are focused on verification of the conception by O. Kernberg dealing with the relationship between dissociative symptoms severity and trauma. Although the conducted research is more and more methodologically correct, certain details still need polishing up so that decisive findings could be obtained in issues of interest.

CHAPTER SEVEN

DISSOCIATION IN BORDERLINE PERSONALITY DISORDER[1]

MARILYN I KORZEKWA AND PAUL F. DELL

Introduction

Borderline Personality Disorder (BPD) is a serious mental health problem, affecting approximately 0.7 - 1.8% of the population (Torgersen, Kringlen, & Cramer, 2001; Swartz et al., 1990) and up to 23% of outpatients (Korzekwa et al., 2008). According to the Diagnostic and Statistical Manual of Mental Disorders, Fourth Edition (DSM-IV; American Psychiatric Association [APA], 1994), symptoms include 5 of 9 of the following: frantic efforts to avoid abandonment, unstable and intense interpersonal relationships, an unstable sense of self, impulsive self-damaging behaviours, recurrent self-mutilating behaviours or suicide attempts, affective instability, a chronic sense of emptiness, inappropriate anger, and stress-related paranoia or severe dissociation. These clients suffer emotionally, their relationships are chaotic, and their self-mutilating (found in 63%) and suicidal behaviours (70%) can be life-threatening (Gunderson, 1994). Indeed, the completed suicide rate is about 10% (Paris & Zweig-Frank, 2001).

The ninth diagnostic criterion for BPD was added to the DSM-IV in 1994, "transient, stress-related paranoid ideation or severe dissociative symptoms" (APA, 1994) because research showed that dissociative symptoms are highly specific for BPD as compared to other psychiatric diagnoses (Gunderson, Zanarini & Kisiel, 1991).

Definitions of Dissociation

Dissociation is defined in the DSM-IV as "a disruption of the usually integrated functions of consciousness, memory, identity or perception of the environment" (APA, 1994). "Normal" dissociative experiences are distributed normally in the population and include intense absorption in tasks such as movies or driving; daydreaming; or infrequent, brief, trauma-related feelings that the world around one seems unreal (derealization) or that one's body or feelings seem unreal (depersonalization) or time-distorted.

Dissociation is pathological when it is not precipitated by stress, occurs frequently and produces distress or dysfunction (Steinberg, 1994). In addition to pathological derealization and depersonalization, other pathological dissociative symptoms include amnesia for personal information or events that are too extensive to be explained by ordinary forgetfulness (dissociative amnesia) and finding evidence of activity of dissociated ego states or alternate identities among possessions or in new talents, by learning from others about times when one acted like a different person, feeling possessed or controlled, and experiencing internal images and voices (identity alteration). Pathological dissociative experiences are distributed categorically in the population, and when severe, are characteristic of a dissociative disorder (Waller, Putnam & Carlson, 1996).

A dissociated ego state is defined as an "internal structure" that operates separately from the person's conscious mind; it "contains" disowned aspects of self or others. A person with a dissociated ego state experiences 1. recurrent intrusive experiences (e.g., feelings, impulses, actions, and thoughts) that are perceived as "not me" - that is, as abnormal, not explained as delusional -, and are a source of distress or dysfunction; 2. recurrent amnesia; and 3. loss or alteration of identity or self (Dell, 2009).

DSM-IV Dissociative Disorders (DDs) include Dissociative Amnesia (DA), Dissociative Fugue, Depersonalization Disorder (DPD), Dissociative Disorder Not Otherwise Specified (DDNOS), and Dissociative Identity Disorder (DID). The diagnostic criteria for DID, formerly known as Multiple Personality Disorder, require 1. the presence of two or more distinct identities or personality states; 2. at least two of these identities or personality states recurrently taking control of the person's behaviour; and 3. dissociative amnesia. Type 1 DDNOS is described as "clinical presentations similar to DID that fail to meet full criteria for the disorder" (APA, 1994). In the general population, the prevalence of DDs and DID is about 10% and 1%, respectively. In psychiatric inpatients, the rates of DDs and DID are about 16% and 4% (Ross, Duffy & Ellason, 2002).

Dissociation is most commonly measured using the Dissociative Experiences Scale (DES), a 28-item self-report questionnaire that rates the frequency (from 0-100% of the time) of experiences of derealization, depersonalization, amnesia, identity alteration, déjà vu and absorption (Carlson & Putnam, 1993). The DES is a screening instrument; it measures normal and pathological dissociative experiences (Waller, Putnam, & Carlson, 1996), does not comprehensively measure the domain of pathological dissociation (Dell, 2006), and does not make DD diagnoses. "Normals" generally score below 10; anxiety, affective and psychotic disorders between 10-18; and Post-Traumatic Stress Disorder (PTSD), DA, and DPD score between 20-30. Scores of 30 or greater should be followed up with a structured clinical interview (Carlson & Putnam, 1993).

The Multidimensional Inventory of Dissociation (MID) is a 218 item self-report questionnaire that diagnoses dissociative disorders, measures 23 manifestations of dissociation, has five validity scales (defensiveness, bizarre symptoms, emotional suffering, attention-seeking, and factitiousness) and has a BPD index. The MID has demonstrated high correlations with trauma history and with other dissociation instruments (Dell, 2006).

Administering the Structured Clinical Interview for DSM-IV Dissociative Disorders-Revised (SCID-D-R) (Steinberg, 1994) is the most reliable method of measuring the severity of dissociation and diagnosing DSM-IV DDs. The SCID-D-R must be administered by a clinician who is experienced in diagnosing dissociative disorders.

Dissociation in BPD: Literature Review

DES scores in BPD averaged 23.7 (range 19-44) across 14 studies that included 880 subjects [2]. DES scores are consistently significantly higher in BPD than controls (normals, other personality disorders, and general psychiatric patients; Herman, Perry, & Van der Kolk, 1989; Ross, 2007; Simeon et al., 2003; Zanarini et al., 2000). BPD patients with high DES scores have a mixture of normal and pathological dissociation (Goodman et al., 2003).

Zanarini used the DES to look at dissociative subgroups in 290 BPD inpatients (diagnosed by the structured interview; Zanarini et al., 2000). Thirty-two percent of the sample could be placed in the low dissociation group (DES scores 1-10), 42% in the moderate dissociation group (scores of 10-29.9), and 26% in the high dissociation group (scores greater than 30).

Laddis and Dell examined 30 BPD subjects (diagnosed by the structured interview) with the MID. They were able to divide them into four subgroups: 1. BPD with no DD (30%). These subjects exhibited some flashbacks, but no voices, and no dissociated ego-states; 2. BPD with dissociative symptoms (30%). These subjects experienced strong flashbacks, memory problems but little frank amnesia, trance, and angry dissociated ego states; 3. BPD with DDNOS (13%). These subjects described strong flashbacks, "coming to" from amnesia experiences, internal voices, and child and persecutor dissociated ego-states; and 4. BPD with DID (27%). These subjects met all DSM-IV DID criteria. (Laddis & Dell, 2002)

Only a handful of studies have rigorously applied DSM-IV Dissociative Disorders criteria in well-diagnosed BPD subjects. Sar et al. (2006) administered the SCID-D-R to 80 randomly-selected university students with BPD and found that 12.5% had Dissociative Amnesia,7.5% Depersonalization Disorder, 42.5% DDNOS, and 10% DID. In another study, Sar et al. (2003) screened psychiatric outpatients with the DES, the SDQ, and DSM-III-R BPD criteria and followed up high scorers with a SCID-D interview. Of 25 BPD patients, 4% were diagnosed with comorbid DA, 36% DDNOS, and 24% DID. In summary, the prevalence of 'no dissociative disorder' in BPD clinical and non-clinical populations varies from 25-35%. The prevalence of DID is about 10-25%. The remainder of BPD subjects, "the middle group", has a variety of dissociative pathologies that meet criteria for a dissociative disorder.

Especially concerning are the findings that BPD patients with high dissociation compared to those with low dissociation have more: suicide attempts, self-injurious behaviour (SIB), analgesia for SIB; global psychopathology; depression; behavioural problems, and use of psychiatric services (Brodsky, Cloitre, & Dulit, 1995; Russ et al., 1993; Shearer, 1994).

Our Research

The objectives of our research are to (1) thoroughly diagnose BPD and dissociative disorders, (2) provide a comprehensive description of the dissociative symptoms that occur in BPD, and (3) compare diagnostic subgroups in terms of their possible etiological factors, comorbid diagnoses, self-harm, and suicidality (Korzekwa et al., 2009). Exclusion criteria included illiteracy, active substance abuse, psychosis and organic disorder. We utilized the Structured Clinical Interview for Axis I Disorders (SCID-I) and self-report for Axis II disorders (SCID-II), the self-report DES, MID, and Childhood Trauma Questionnaire (Bernstein & Fink, 1998), and the SCID-D-R interview. The inter-rater reliability on the SCID-D-R was checked via videotape ratings by an independent expert (intra-class coefficient = 0.71).

In Study 1, we screened our entire general outpatient psychiatric clinic (n=360) in order to obtain cross-sectional prevalence data on BPD. We diagnosed BPD in 54 of the clinic patients (on the structured interview; Korzekwa et al., 2008), 21 of whom completed the dissociation portion of the study. Among those 21 BPD patients, 23.8% had no DD, 9.5% Dissociative Amnesia, 19% Depersonalization Disorder, 23.8% DDNOS, and 23.8% DID. Most of the 21 BPD patients (86%) had a current mood disorder (62% had depression and 24% bipolar affective disorder). Our BPD sample averaged an astounding 3.3 anxiety disorders per patient (i.e., 86% had PTSD. 76% panic disorder, 57% social phobia, 52% generalized anxiety disorder, 43% obsessive compulsive disorder, and 19% a specific phobia). Our 86% rate of PTSD is strikingly high, probably because a majority of our patients had been referred from inpatient or emergency services.

In Study 2, we invited consecutive new admissions to our day-hospital to participate. To date, we have collected dissociation data on nine additional persons with BPD. The combined sample of 30 BPD subjects was 80% female. The average age was 35.2 (*SD* = 9.0); 60% had never been married and 23.4% had never worked. The 30 BPD patients averaged 13.1 (*SD* = 2.3) years of education (most had completed secondary school); they averaged 3.4 (*SD* = 6.5) lifetime hospitalizations.

The most frequent SCID-D-R symptoms in the combined sample are listed in Table 1. Frequency of dissociative symptoms appears to lie upon a spectrum of increasing severity of DD diagnosis. Especially surprising is the fact that dissociative symptoms were frequent, even in BPD patients without a comorbid DD (or with only a "mild DD" such as DA and DPD).

Table 7-1. Frequency of SCID-D-R symptoms in 30 BPD patients

Frequency of Symptom (%)	No DD (N=7) (%)	DA, DPD (n=10) (%)	DDNOS, DID (n=13) (%)	Total (n=30) (%)
Depersonalization: Watching self from outside the body	29	60	92	67
Going through motions, real self seems to be far away	0	70	77	57
Feel like 2 people, one observing and one participating	29	30	77	50
One's self or body feels unreal	0	20	54	30
Feel like a stranger to oneself	14	20	62	37
Not in control of emotions	57	60	85	70
Not in control of behaviour	29	30	92	57
Not in control of speech	0	20	69	37
Derealization: Surroundings, other people feel unreal	14	20	46	30
Puzzled about what is real and not real in surroundings	14	20	38	27
Amnesia: Large memory gaps	29	20	69	43
Amnesia for daily activities	0	30	77	40
Finding oneself somewhere, no memory of going there	0	20	69	37
Amnesia for personal information	0	10	46	23
Identity Alteration: Acting like a different person	14	0	69	33
Acting like a child	0	20	46	27
Hearing voices inside the head	14	40	46	37
Hearing voices outside the head	29	0	38	23
Derealization: Surroundings, other people feel unreal	0	20	54	30

To determine the dissociative symptoms of the average BPD patient, we constructed a list of the MID dissociation items that were endorsed at a clinically significant level by at least 50% of our subjects:

-amnesia for recent and remote events and large memory gaps
-memory blackouts or blank spells
-"coming to" in the middle of a conversation with no memory of what was said
-being bothered by how much they were forgetting
-forgetting causing difficulties for them
-difficulty remembering daily activities, such as whether they had eaten
-they did or said things when they were angry that they did not remember
-they were bothered by how frequently and suddenly they found themselves in a trance
-people noticed their "being gone"
-other people think that they live in a world of their own
-they often felt different from themselves and did not feel "together" or "whole"
-frequent derealization and feeling "disconnected"
-puzzled about what is real and what is not real in their environment
-they heard internal voices that were telling them to "shut up"
-they experienced thoughts as being inserted into their mind
-they felt that strong emotions like hurt or anger "came from out of nowhere"
-people told them that at times they acted so differently that they seemed like another person
-vivid and sudden or uncontrolled flashbacks experienced in all senses
-flashback which lasted for days, and resulted in loss of contact with the present
-they were so bothered by the flashbacks that they found it hard to get out of bed or function at work
-the flashbacks made them want to inflict pain on themselves or die.

Table 7-2 examines dissociative severity (the four SCID-D-R subgroups) as a function of possible etiologic factors, comorbid diagnoses, self-harm, and suicidality. Strong associations of DD with flashbacks, and childhood sexual and total abuse are consistent with current etiological theories (see below). Associations of dissociative severity with a number of current anxiety disorders and current general axis I disorders are new and noteworthy findings. The association of dissociative severity with the MID self-harm scale, (which includes items such as hearing a voice inside your head that wants you to die or to hurt yourself, having traumatic flashbacks that make you want to inflict pain on yourself, and nobody understands how much you hurt) is of especial concern. We expect that these associations would be clinically significant with a larger sample size.

Table 7-2. ANOVA comparison of the four SCID-D-R subgroups in terms of possible etiologic factors, comorbid diagnoses and self-harm.

Four SCID-D-R Subgroups: No DD; DA or DPD; DDNOS type 1; DID	
Significant or strong trend ANOVA Tests	p values
Number of current anxiety disorders	.005
MID Flashbacks scale	.016
Childhood Sexual Abuse	.017
Number of current Axis I disorders	.021
Total Childhood Trauma	.030
Childhood Emotional Neglect	.071
MID Self-Harm scale	.079

Neurobiology of Dissociation in BPD

The generally accepted understanding of the mechanism of brain pathology in BPD is that the prefrontal cortex (PFC) fails to inhibit excessive amygdale activation (Tebartz van Elst et al., 2003). The amygdale's role is to evaluate the threat potential of events and determine the emotional reaction. Hyper-reactivity of the amygdala in BPD has been demonstrated in several functional MRI studies of responses to emotional stimuli (Donegan et al., 2003) and there is evidence that there are abnormalities in the PFC microstructure (Rusch et al., 2007). In dissociation, however, the autonomic system is hypo-aroused. For example, in PTSD, 30% of subjects when reading the script of their trauma during neuroimaging will show a dissociated, numb response with lack of heart rate increase. Their FMRI scans show a pattern of increased activity in the PFC areas and anterior cingulate cortex (which regulates the autonomic, neuroendocrine and behavioural aspects of emotional response), but without increased activation of the amygdala (Lanius et al., 2005). According to the "cortico-limbic model of dissociation" (Sierra & Berrios, 1998), this pattern is thought to represent enhanced suppression by the prefrontal areas of fear-induced arousal. The function of this mechanism is to turn off the unbearable panic, or as a freezing/helpless response. It is probably mediated by the dorsal vagal parasympathetic system. (Frewen & Lanius, 2006).

In BPD, the cortico-limbic model of dissociation is evident in startle response studies, where high dissociators (compared to low dissociators) have a blunted startle response (as measured by an electromyogram [Ebner-Priemer et al., 2005]). The startle response is mainly mediated by the amygdala. Further evidence of this model is found in BPD subjects with self-injurious behaviour (SIB). High dissociators compared to low dissociators have more analgesia with SIB, higher pain thresholds, and less brain activity (fMRI) in response to identical heat stimuli. This represents cortical suppression of sensory (pain) information (Schmahl et al., 2006).

When subjects with both BPD and dissociative disorders (diagnosed by SCID-D-R) are studied, their brain scans are more consistent with scans found in depersonalization disorder (Simeon et al., 2000) and DID (Reinders et al., 2006), namely dysfunction of widespread somatosensory integration areas. Lange et al. studied 17 female BPDs with severe childhood sexual and physical abuse histories with the following comorbid DDs: 14 DPD, 4 DA, and 1 DID. They found significant decreases (at rest) of glucose metabolism compared to controls in the left precuneus area of the parietal lobe (consistent with a hypnotic state) and in the right temporal pole (which correlated with impaired memory) as well as other areas of the temporal and parietal cortices (Lange et al., 2005).

Neurotransmitters involved in dissociation in BPD include norepinephrine (lower basal urinary levels [Simeon et al., 2007]), cortisol (greater response to stress [Simeon et al., 2007]), glutamate - NMDA receptor (ketamine; Grosjean & Tsai, 2007), endogenous opioids (Philipsen et al., 2004) and serotonin (Stein et al., 1996). (For a more detailed neurobiological review see Korzekwa, Dell, & Pain, 2009).

Etiology

The aetiology of dissociation is thought to conform to a stress-diathesis interactional model (Dell, 2009). The diathesis is the capacity to dissociate, which is necessary for the development of dissociation and is sometimes sufficient alone to explain dissociation. The capacity for dissociation is largely genetic, being as much as 59% heritable (Becker-Blease et al., 2004) and partly comprised of hypnotisability, which is up to 63% heritable (Morgan, 1973). However, disorganized attachment to the primary caregiving figure is also an important predisposing factor (Ogawa et al., 1997). This insecure pattern of attachment occurs when the parents' behaviour is "frightened or frightening", often due to unresolved parental grief or PTSD. The child's reaction is fear, which activates the attachment system, but the caregiver who is supposed to provide comfort and security is the one that is frightening the child (Main & Hesse, 1990). This results in the breakdown of attachment strategy and a "failure of the integrations of consciousness" in the child-a precursor to the development of dissociation (Liotti, 2002).

Traumatic stress is also necessary but not always sufficient alone to explain the development of dissociation. The types of traumatic stress that are more likely to set off dissociation include sexual abuse, torture or pain, and feelings of helplessness or powerlessness. Dissociation is more likely in females, younger children, and the victims of multiple perpetrators or multiple forms of abuse. Other stressors such as severe neglect and confinement abuse may also lead to dissociation. (Draijer & Langeland, 1999; Ogawa, et al., 1997; Perry et al., 1995).

In BPD, genetic factors also contribute to the capacity to dissociate. These include affect dysregulation (45% heritable; Briere, 2006; Jang et al., 1996) and neurocognitive executive functioning deficits (77% heritable; Judd, 2005). Studies of attachment in BPD reveal that disorganized (called unresolved in adults) attachment is the most common (50-89%), while anxious-preoccupied insecure attachment is also common (23-75%) and secure attachment is rare in BPD (0-8%; Agrawal et al., 2004). In general populations, the pattern is reversed: secure attachment is the most common and disorganized-unresolved is infrequent.

Childhood abuse and trauma is also extremely common in BPD. For example, a recent study of 214 BPD outpatients (Battle et al., 2004) found neglect experiences in 90%, all forms of childhood abuse in 81%, and childhood sexual abuse (CSA) in 44%. Rates of CSA and multiple forms of abuse are greater in BPD than controls in most studies (Herman, Perry, & Van der Kolk, 1989; Laporte & Guttman, 2001; Links et al., 1988). With these high rates of childhood trauma in BPD, one would think that childhood abuse is correlated with dissociation in BPD. This is the case in most simple regression analyses (Herman, Perry, & Van der Kolk, 1989; Goodman et al., 2003; Van Den Bosch et al., 2003) and 4/7 of the multiple regression analyses (Brodsky, Cloitre & Dulit, 1995; Ross-Gower et al., 1998; Shearer, 1994; Zanarini et al., 2000). However, three multiple regression analysis studies found that dissociation in BPD is not significantly related to childhood trauma (Simeon et al., 2003; Zwieg-Frank, Paris & Guzder, 1994a & 1994b). Therefore, it is logical to conclude that there are two groups of BPD patients: (1) BPD patients for whom dissociation is a response to childhood trauma and (2) BPD patients for whom dissociation appears to be mediated by other factors such as neglect, inconsistent treatment by a caregiver, fearful attachment, severe maternal dysfunction, witnessing of violence, sexual assault as an adult, or substance abuse (Shearer, 1994; Simeon et al., 2003; Van Den Bosch et al., 2003; Zanarini et al., 2000). Indeed, substance abusing BPD patients can have dissociation without a trauma history since intoxication effects may be confused with dissociative symptoms (Van Den Bosch et al., 2003).

In summary, Table 7-3 presents a proposed integrated hypothesis of aetiology of dissociation in BPD. Not all BPD patients dissociate. Not all BPD patients who dissociate have been abused. Not all BPD patients have a disorganized attachment status. The key factors in the low and high dissociators are probably the attachment status and the genetic capacity to dissociate. Without the capacity to dissociate, dissociation is unlikely, regardless of trauma "dose". The "middle" group with "mild" dissociation, predominately of the depersonalization type, could arise from several different pathways: anxious attachment with moderate to high trauma and moderate to high capacity for dissociation; anxious attachment and substance abuse; disorganized attachment and another factor such as neglect, witnessing violence or assault as an adult; or disorganized attachment and minimal trauma but moderate to high capacity to dissociate. In DID, all three causative factors are extreme. In DDNOS, one or two of the factors are less extreme than in DID.

Table 7-3. A Proposed Integrated Hypothesis of Etiology

Subtype of BPD	Attachment	Trauma	Capacity to dissociate
None to minimal dissociation (20-30%)	Secure or anxious	None to moderate	Low
Significant de-personalization (10-30%)	Anxious or disorganized	Mild to severe; other factors	Low to high
DDNOS (20-40%)	Disorganized	Moderate to severe	Moderate to high
DID (10-25%)	Disorganized	Severe	High

Assessment and Treatment

We recommend that all BPD patients be screened with the DES. For high scoring or significant pathological dissociation items, the therapist should ask for examples. Intoxication and medical causes (e.g., seizures) should be ruled out. High DES scores should be followed up with the self-report MID or SCID-D-R interview. It is especially important to be aware of the presence of dissociated ego states that may cause self-harm or attempt suicide when dissociated. It is extremely beneficial to form an alliance with angry ego states early in therapy.

Zanarini et al. (2008) examined dissociation in BPD over a 10 year period in 290 subjects, 70% of whom were still receiving therapy at follow-up. In table 4, we see that the overall sample improved from a moderate to a low score and that high dissociators fell to the moderate group and moderate dissociators fell to the low group. Therefore, treatment as usual resulted in the reduction of dissociation to normal levels in the average BPD patient over 10 years. However, 14 subjects from the low and moderate groups had a "new onset" of high dissociation and 18 subjects who had dropped from the high to the moderate group had a "recurrence" of high dissociation during the follow-up period. Together with the 15 subjects who had high dissociation throughout the 10 years, this means that 16% of the total sample had DES profiles that suggest a serious DD that did not improve with treatment as usual.

Table 7- 4. The Course of Dissociation in BPD: 10 Year Follow-up (Zanarini et al., 2008)

DES Group	N (baseline)	DES	
		Baseline	10 years
Low (0-9.9)	92	5.1	3.1
Moderate (10-29.9)	122	17.5	6.8
High (30+)	76	48.4	17.7
Total	290	21.8	8.5

BPD treatment studies where dissociation was treated intentionally as a symptom demonstrate significant reductions in dissociation. In dialectical behaviour therapy, dissociation is labeled as a "problem behaviour", the predisposing events are analyzed, emotion regulation skills are taught, and triggers to past trauma are desensitized. Two randomized controlled trials support the effectiveness of DBT in treating dissociation compared to waitlist or treatment as usual (Koons et al., 2001; Bohus et al., 2004). Cognitive analytic therapy systematically seeks out and describes dissociated states and increases integration by increasing awareness, and control of these states (Wildgoose, Clarke & Waller, 2001). In psychodynamically-oriented trauma-focused treatment, past traumatic memories are processed on an inpatient unit with eye movement desensitization and reprocessing, followed by a psychodynamic working-through that especially works with regressed ego states (Sachsse, Vogel & Leichsenring, 2006).

When the DES was used to assess efficacy of standard BPD treatments, research also showed a significant improvement in DES scores. These treatments included psychoanalytic transference-focused psychotherapy compared to schema-focused therapy (Kremers et al., 2006) and dynamic deconstructive psychotherapy (Gregory et al., 2008).

Medications have not been shown to be effective for treating dissociation in BPD in randomized controlled studies. The only randomized double-blind medication (cross-over design) study found equal reductions of dissociation with both Naloxone (opiate receptor antagonist) and placebo in nine BPD subjects with SIB with analgesia (Philipsen, Schmahl & Lieb, 2004).

In summary, evidence based treatments for BPD result in improved dissociation in low and moderate dissociators. Treatments that teach emotion awareness and emotion regulation, and trauma-cue desensitization are more effective than treatments as usual. However, high dissociators require a more complex three-phase treatment: 1. a stabilization phase that may last months to years and starts with BPD treatments but adds techniques such as education about trauma and dissociation, ego strength building, containment of trauma memories through imagery, "grounding" skills (i.e., being present in the moment), safety planning, and working through re-enactments; 2. a trauma processing phase where the goal is to desensitize the traumatic affect and restructure traumatic personal schemas. With highly dissociative clients, trauma processing requires specialized training; and 3. an integration-rehabilitation phase that focuses on consolidation of gains (Chu, 1998; ISSD, 2005).

Conclusions

The DSM-IV "does not provide an adequate description of the dissociative comorbidity in BPD" (Ross, 2007, p. 79). Dissociation is very common in BPD and is more common in BPD than other personality disorders and non-DD clients, but dissociation is not an inherent aspect of BPD. Although BPD clients report significantly more childhood abuse that most non-DD psychiatric clients, some BPD patients in the low and moderate dissociation groups do not have childhood abuse histories. Other factors which may be involved include substance abuse, disorganized attachment, the inheritance of BPD traits and the capacity for dissociation, dysfunctional frontal-limbic pathways, and over-endorsing of symptoms due to emotional suffering and attention seeking.

All BPD patients should be screened with the DES. High scores should be followed-up with detailed inquiry or structured assessment (MID or SCID-D-R). Clients with low to moderate dissociation scores are expected to improve with treatments that assess and treat dissociation as a symptom and teach understanding and regulation of emotion. High dissociators are at higher risk for SIB, suicide attempts, and hospitalization; and require more complex treatments.

20-30% of BPD patients have dissociation scores in the normal range. They likely have secure or insecure-anxious attachment status and a low genetic capacity for dissociating. Amygdala activity is excessive and poorly inhibited by the prefrontal cortex.

40-60% of BPD patients have moderate dissociation scores. In our research they had frequent, lengthy and stress-related depersonalization and amnesia; some dissociated ego states. Their attachment status is probably anxious or disorganized; severity of trauma (which can be mild to severe), interacts with the capacity to dissociate (which can be low to high). Non-trauma factors may play a role in aetiology. Startle response and pain tolerance studies show cortical suppression of limbic emotional activity and brain imaging shows a widespread somatosensory lack of integration. Their dissociation symptoms respond to the usual BPD treatments, but more rapidly to therapies focused on dissociation and emotion regulation. A subset will still need trauma work.

About 10-25% of BPD patients have comorbid DID. BPD-DID cases in our research had the most frequent, longest duration, and most severe dissociative symptoms. They probably have a high genetic capacity for dissociating and a disorganized-unresolved attachment status. They usually have a severe childhood trauma history. They have dysfunction of widespread somatosensory integration areas of the brain. These extremely ill clients require a complex three-phase therapy.

Notes

[1] Acknowledgements: This study was partially funded by the Department of Psychiatry and Behavioural Neurosciences at McMaster University. Earlier versions of this work were presented at the 23rd and 25th annual conferences of the International Society for the Study of Trauma and Dissociation, 2006 & 2008, Los Angeles and Chicago, USA, and the Association for Research in Personality Disorders, annual meeting 2009, San Francisco, USA.

[2] Meta-analysis was performed by the first author; a complete list of references is available from author.

CHAPTER EIGHT

THE NOTION OF TRAUMA AND REVICTIMISATION IN AN ANALYSIS OF THE BEHAVIOUR OF PEOPLE WITH A PSYCHOPATHIC PERSONALITY STRUCTURE

BEATA PASTWA-WOJCIECHOWSKA

Introduction

Individuals of a psychopathic personality structure are mostly associated with acts of aggression and violence that they inflict on others. It is hard to disagree with this image since the clinical description of psychopathic personality seems to confirm such observations. In the eyes of the public, psychopaths are also considered to be dominated by aggression and violence. Therefore, we should ask whether the aetiology and development of this disorder can be analysed in the context of experiencing traumatic events. Such a question may appear to be tricky, as the literature definition of aggression describes it as a learned form of behaviour. How learning becomes a way of acquiring and demonstrating aggressive behaviour is explained by A.H. Buss (1962) in the behaviouristic approach and A. Bandura (1973) in the convention of social learning. On the other hand, the concepts of aggression accentuating its adapting role (Leary, 1957; Stanik, 1980) bring attention to the fact that aggressive forms of interpersonal behaviour are oriented on adapting a person to their surroundings, which means the reduction of anxiety and the creation of a feeling of dignity. Recent studies into the psychopathic personality show irrefutably that psychopaths themselves often experienced violence in childhood (Pastwa-Wojciechowska, 2010). Especially emphasised here is the role of studies into the structure of family, of its functions fulfilled by its members and methods of upbringing used in the process of socialisation of psychopathic people (Ostrowska, 19981, Gierowski et al., 1996, Pastwa-Wojciechowska, 2004, 2010). In other words, irrespective of the research perspective or paradigm, the results of the studies irrefutably indicate the occurrence of a relationship between experiencing harm and later demonstrating aggressive behaviour, which in extreme cases can assume the form of criminal behaviour.

In analysing the influence of victimisation on criminal behaviour, many authors (Widom, Ames, 1994; Hamilton-Giachritsis et al., 2005; Odgers et al., 2005) underline that the experience of harm and/or neglect is connected with a later tendency to undertake criminal forms of behaviour. At the same time, it is noted that children experience several forms of harm concurrently, and determining the influence of individual types of harm is unusually difficult. One cannot, however, stress enough that, based on prospective studies, estimates are that one in six children who are victims of physical abuse will in the future become abusers themselves (Widom, 1991; Hamilton-Giachritsis et al., 2005) and one in five abused sexually will later commit sexual crimes (Hamilton-Giachritsis et al., 2005). Therefore, in view of these studies, it seems important not to perceive all harmed children as a homogenous group, but carefully and objectively analyse factors that can contribute to the victim-offender cycle. I would like to define the notions of victimisation and revictimisation, which are key terms in this article. As a starting point, I would like to suggest the terminology developed by Hamilton and Browne (1998) referring to various patterns of individual and repeated acts of harm, who distinguish between 1) individual victimisation, that is, a single act of harm committed by only one offender - a member of the family or another person; 2) multiple victimisation - a single act of harm committed by more than one offender - the offenders may be members of the family or other people; 3) repeated victimisation - harm done at least twice by the same offender(s) - a member of the family or another person; 4) revictimisation - harm done at least twice by various offenders. It is worth noting that in the Polish practice of the justice system, victimisation is defined as that moment of committing a crime when the victim is harmed for the first time. The notion of revictimisation is identified with repeated victimisation (harm).

In ordering the terminological confusion prevailing in clinical terminology, I would like to emphasise that in this article the notion of psychopathy will be defined in line with the operational concept of psychopathy by Robert D. Hare (1991/2002), and the method of diagnosing psychopathy - *The Psychopathy Checklist-Revised* (PCL-R). The criteria of diagnosis suggested by Hare (1991/2002) allow for the measurement of two factors, while each of them is described by 10 items. Thus, factor one describes a constellation of psychopathic traits considered by many clinicists to be basic for this type of personality, that is, factors concerning interpersonal, emotional and verbal styles of functioning [1) Glib and superficial charm, 2) Grandiose estimation of self, 3) Increased need for stimulation and increased susceptibility to boredom, 4) Pathological lying, 5) Pursuit of leadership by manipulation, 6) Lack of remorse or guilt, 7) Shallow affect, 8) Callousness and lack of empathy, 9) Parasitic lifestyle, 10) Poor behavioural controls]. This factor correlates positively with clinical determinants of psychopathy, especially with narcissistic and histrionic personality disorders and measures of Machiavellianism. On the other hand, it correlates negatively with the measures of empathy and fear. Factor two describes types of behaviour indicating impulsiveness, lack of stability and antisocial lifestyle: [11) Sexual promiscuity, 12) Early behaviour problems, 13) Lack of realistic, long-term goals, 14) Impulsiveness, 15) Irresponsibility, recklessness, 16) Failure to accept responsibility for one's own actions, 17) Many, short-term relationships, 18) Juvenile delinquency, 19) Revocation of conditional release, 20) Criminal versatility]. Variables contained in this factor correlate with the criteria of antisocial personality disorders (Hare, 1991/2002). In analysing the variables with regard to their meaning for the process of self-regulation and self-control we can group them into those considered significant (axial) for this type of personality, and those that lead to certain effects and consequences resulting from them.

Generally, the conducted studies have aimed at a clinical and empirical analysis of the effects of a trauma experienced in early childhood by people with a psychopathic personality structure. At the same time they attempted to determine possible types of victimisation experienced by the participants. The intensity of psychopathic traits was evaluated according to formal and content criteria described in the Psychopathy Checklist-Revised (PCL-R), simultaneously defining the variable as a dependent one.The notions of trauma, traumatic experience and type of victimisation were treated as independent variables. The studies also traced the relation between sex and the personality structure of the participants, and the type and frequency of experienced traumatic events. According to the presented assumptions, a thorough analysis covered:- type and frequency of traumatic experiences in early childhood in people with a psychopathic personality structure,- the occurrence of diversification of traumatic experiences in early childhood in the groups with regard to sex,- type of victimisation experienced by the participants,- relation between the structure of psychopathy and type and frequency of traumatic events experienced by the participants.

In other words, based on the issues presented above, the following study questions were posed:1) What early childhood traumatic events are the most common among the participants?2) Does sex diversify the frequency of experiencing traumatic event or events in the participants?3) What kind of victimisation was experienced by the participants?4) Is there a relation between the structure of psychopathy and type and frequency of traumatic events experienced by the participants?

Study participants

The studies covered a total of 60 people. According to the study problems presented above, the following criteria of selecting the participants were used: 1) a legally binding conviction, 2) serving a prison sentence, 3) age - above 18 years old (according to the diagnostic criteria of DSM and ICD), 4) psychiatric, or psychiatric and psychological diagnosis of dissociative personality disorders, 5) a result obtained in the Psychopathy Checklist-Revised (PCL-R) equaling or exceeding 30 points, 6) sex - men and women. Considering the above criteria two equal groups were formed (N=30), and the analysis used the ANOVA method: 2x(2) - Sex x PCL-R Scale with a repeated measurement within the PCL-R Scale factor. Thus, it was concluded that there was a statistically significant and important difference between men and women with regard to psychopathic intensity ($F(1;58)=79.01$, $p<0.001$, Eta2=0.58), where male participants showed a greater intensity of psychopathic traits.

The average age of the female participants was 33 years (SD=3.2; min. 28, max. 39), while the average age of male participants was 30 years (SD= 2.2; min. 24, max. 43). A comparison between the groups using the Student's t-test for independent samples indicated statistically significant differences of age averages [$t(58)=-4.55$; $p<0.001$].

Study methods

The methods served to operationalise the following variables: (1) psychopathic personality, (2) structure of psychopathy, (3) traumatic factors and (4) course and type of victimisation.

In order to verify empirically the variables, the following study methods were used:

1. The Psychopathy Checklist-Revised (PCL-R) by Robert D. Hare in the Polish adaptation by B. Pastwa-Wojciechowska (2004). The method allows for three measurements: a) an evaluation of psychopathic traits intensity (general result), b) an evaluation of clinical traits of psychopathy within the emotional and interpersonal dimension (Factor 1) and c) behavioural indicators of behaviour characteristics for psychopathy (Factor 2). Each of the twenty items in PCL-R is spread over a three-point scale (0, 1, 2). Assigning a given item 0 points means that it does not refer to a participant or show traits or behaviour described in the item, or presents a description other than the one contained in the item, or one that is incoherent with the item's description. One (1) point is assigned when the item refers to the participant to some extent, but does not fulfill all the requirements necessary to be given 2 points. In other words, some estimations match, but there are too many exceptions or doubts to give 2 points, or when a given item refers to the item in a way unspecified in the administration of the test or there is a discrepancy between the information collected during an interview and data in the files, which makes it impossible to assign either 2 or 0 points. Two (2) points are given for an item, when all requirements are fully met and all necessary comparisons (estimations) are accepted, and the behaviour of a participant fully corresponds to the intention and description of the item.

2. Lifetime Trauma and Victimization History (LTVH) C.S. Widom, M.A. Dutton, S.J. Czaja, and K.A. DuMont (2005) in the Polish adaptation by B. Pastwa-Wojciechowska. The questionnaire contains 30 life events referring to traumatic experiences and the course of victimisation, on which the participants comment. The information is obtained from various sources - mostly based on a structured conversation and interview with participants, analysis of court files and interviews of various people and organisations (institutions). It is assumed that in this method, an interview is the basis of systematic and exhaustive acquirement of information concerning traumatic life events and experiences of victimisation. It also includes such factors as age of a participant, time of an event, relationship with an offender, an evaluation of threat, and frequency of described events. The questionnaire specifies stressors regardless of symptoms. Moreover, the stressors included in the test are grouped into seven categories (general trauma, physical assault/abuse, sexual assault/abuse, family/friend murdered or committed suicide, witnessing a trauma by someone else, criminal victimisations, and kidnapping/stalking).

Organisation of studies

The planned study procedure required the inclusion of a clinical criterion, that is, psychopathic personality disorders, as well as a legal criterion connected with the breach of legal rules. Therefore, the concentration of there two variables required planning of the studies in such a way that a series of demographic, psychopathologic and criminological factors could be controlled. All participants were studied individually and they gave direct consent for the studies to be performed. Consent was also obtained from the directors of penitentiary facilities in which the participants were located. After selecting the participants with regard to psychiatric or psychiatric and psychological diagnosis, both in the court proceedings and under conditions of incarceration, a study using the Psychopathy Checklist-Revised test was conducted, allowing us to confirm, according to the concept of R. Hare (1991/2002), whether or not the participants had psychopathic personality structures. Then the participants answered questions included in the Lifetime Trauma and Victimization History questionnaire, concerning their possible traumatic experiences in early childhood.

Results

Below, according to the presented purposes of the studies, their results are shown.

Traumatic experiences in early childhood

At the beginning it was analysed which early childhood traumatic events were the most common among the participants (Table 8-1).

The studies revealed that among 30 listed traumatic events evaluated with the Lifetime Trauma and Victimization History questionnaire by C.S Wodom et al., in a Polish adaptation by B. Pastwa-Wojciechowska, the participants enumerated 16 events (53%) as being those they encountered, while 14 (47%) events were not experienced by any of the participants. Thus, most often the participants came into contact with the following traumatic events: being face to face with danger (57%), physical injury in childhood (55%), seeing another person with physical injuries (38%), physical injury (32%), sexual abuse in childhood (25%), stealing without the use of violence (25%), a threat of firearm use (22%), witnessing a sexual assault on another person (20%), a member of their family or a friend being murdered (18%), a serious accident (15%), stealing with the

Table 8-1 Type and number of experienced traumatic events in the studied group of men and women in the Lifetime Trauma and Victimization History questionnaire

Study variables	Women Number of events (N)	Men Number of events (N)	Total Number of events (N)
5. Serious accident	3	6	9
7. Physical injury	17	2	19
8. A threat of using a firearm	5	11	16
9. Being face to face with danger	15	21	36
11. Physical harm in childhood	17	17	34
12. Sexual abuse in childhood	6	0	6
16. A member of family/friend being murdered	4	7	11
17. Witnessing a murder or serious bodily injury	2	5	7
18. Witnessing a member of family or a friend commit suicide	0	3	3
20. Seeing another person with physical injuries	23	0	23
21. Witnessing a sexual assault on another person	4	8	12
22. Property damage	2	0	2
23. Stealing with the use of violence	9	0	9
24. Attempted theft with the use of violence	7	0	7
27. Stealing without the use of violence	15	0	15

use of violence (15%), witnessing a murder or serious bodily injury (12%), attempted theft with the use of violence (12%), forced sexual activity (10%), witnessing a family member commit suicide (5%), and property damage (3%). None of the participants indicated any of the following events as a traumatic experience they encountered or did not experience: a natural disaster, a man-made disaster, direct experience of combat (violence), living in a war zone, exposure to a dangerous chemical substance, sexual abuse with a threat of use of a weapon, attempted coercion into sexual activity, invasion of privacy, exposure to a dead body, burglary (in the past), burglary (in the present), kidnapping, stalking, other dangerous situations.

Sex and the frequency of experiencing traumatic events among the participants

Next it was analysed whether sex diversifies the frequency of experiencing a traumatic event or events in the participants (Table 8-1,8- 2).

Table 8-2 Results of a comparison of the number of experienced traumatic events in men and women based on the Lifetime Trauma and Victimization History questionnaire

Traumatic event	Women M (SD)	Men M (SD)	Tests of differences significance
7. Physical injury	0.57 (0.50)	0.07 (0.25)	t=4.853, df=42.81, p<0.001
9. Being face to face with danger	0.43 (0.50)	0.70 (0.47)	t=2.128, df=57.65, p<0.05
10. Sexual abuse in childhood	0.50 (0.51)	0.00 (0.00)	t=5.385, df=29, p<0.001
20. Seeing another person with physical injuries	0.77 (0.43)	0.00 (0.00)	t=9.761, df=29, p<0.001
21. Stealing without the use of violence	0.50 (0.51)	0.00 (0.00)	t=5.385, df=29, p<0.001

A statistical analysis of the student's t-test results for independent samples conducted for the studied traumatic events showed that there are statistically significant differences with regard to the traumatic events between men and women of a psychopathic personality structure (Table 8-2). Thus, the events diversifying the frequency of traumatic events in the groups were physical injury, sexual abuse in childhood, seeing another person with physical injuries and stealing without the use of violence. The women experienced more often such traumatic events as physical injury, sexual abuse in childhood, seeing another person being physically injured and stealing without the use of violence. The men, on the other hand, more often came face to face with danger. It is interesting that men more often than women stated that they felt threatened with the use of a firearm against them, experienced physical injury in childhood and witnessed a sexual assault on another person. The results of the statistical analysis revealed that the differences between men and women are not only statistically significant, but also considerable, which is indicated by a Cohen's d value higher than 0.40. In studying the differences between the groups, it was found that only women experienced such traumatic events diversifying both groups as seeing another person with physical injuries, experiencing sexual abuse in childhood, and stealing without the use of violence.

In a later part of the study, the analysis of frequency of experiencing traumatic events by men and women with a psychopathic personality (Table 8-3) was conducted.

Table 8-3 Frequency of traumatic events experienced by men and women

	Frequency of traumatic events	Total							
	1	2	3	4	5	6	7	10	
Women	0	3	4	8	6	5	3	1	30
	0.00%	10.00%	13.33%	26.67%	20.00%	16.67%	10.00%	3.33%	100%
Men	5	8	12	5	0	0	0	0	30
	16.67%	26.67%	40.00%	16.67%	0.00%	0.00%	0.00%	0.00%	100%
Total	5	11	16	13	6	5	3	1	60
	8.33%	18.33%	26,67%	21.67%	10.00%	8.33%	5.00%	1.67%	100%

Results of the Mann-Whitney test indicate that the difference between men and women with regard to experiencing trauma is statistically significant ($Z=4.767$; $p<0.001$), and on average men ($M=2.57$; $SD=0.97$) experience a smaller number of traumatic events than women ($M=4.70$; $SD=1.76$).

Type of victimisation experienced

Referring to an analysis of the victimisation type experienced by the participants (Table 8-4) it was found that female participants experienced the following types of victimisation:3 (10%) people encountered multiple victimisation (a single act of harm committed by more than one offender), 8 (27%) people experienced repeated victimisation (harm done at least twice by the same offender[s]), 4 (13%) people encountered revictimisation (harm done at least twice by various offenders) and 15 (50%) were faced with repeated victimisation and revictimisation. Among the male participants, 5 (17%) experienced individual victimisation (a single act of harm committed by one offender), 6 (20%) experienced multiple victimisation, 12 (40%) had to deal with repeated victimisation, 2 (6%) encountered revictimisation and 5 (17%) dealt with repeated victimisation and revictimisation.

Table 8-4 Experiencing harm in the study groups

Type of victimisation	Women N	Men N
No victimisation	0	0
Individual victimisation	0	5
Multiple victimisation	3	8
Repeated victimisation	8	12
Revictimisation	4	2
Repeated victimisation or revictimisation	15	5

Relationship between the structure of psychopathy and the type of traumatic experience

In answer to the study question if there is a relationship between the structure of psychopathy and the frequency and type of traumatic experiences encountered by the participants, it was concluded that such a relationship occurs only with Factor I (emotional and interpersonal) of the PCL-R.

As can be seen in Table 8-5, there was a statistically significant relation with seven out of sixteen traumatic events enumerated by the participants, that is, physical injury, a threat of using a firearm, physical abuse in childhood, seeing another person with physical injuries, stealing with the use of violence, attempted theft with the use of violence, and stealing without the use of violence. Interestingly, it can be observed that the calculated relations are negative correlations; that is, in people experiencing a given type of trauma the result for factor I of the PCL-R questionnaire is lower than for people who do not experience the trauma. A different relationship is observed only for the emotional and interpersonal factor and a firearm threat, while an experience of such trauma is connected with a lower PCL-R result in the emotional and interpersonal factor. It should be underlined here that the analysis considered only those events that were indicated by at least three participants. Rarer events were rejected, assuming that they would bring no or a false conclusion of little statistical significance. Factor I of PCL-R showed also a statistically significant relation with the general number of traumatic events experienced by the participants.

Table 8-5 Matrix of correlation between the PCL-R factors and type of experienced traumatic events based on the Lifetime Trauma and Victimization History questionnaire

Event	7. Physical injury	8. Firearm threat	10. Sexual abuse in childhood	20. Seeing a physical injury in another person	23. Stealing with the use of violence	24. Attempted theft with the use of violence	27. Stealing without the use of violence	Number of traumas
Factor I(emotional and interpersonal)	-0.51	0.27	-0.57	-0.61	-0.37	-0.40	-0.57	-0.57

Discussion

The purpose of the study was to evaluate retrospective memories of traumatic events experienced by people with a psychopathic personality structure. First of all, the focus was on the characteristics of traumatic events experienced by the participants. The psychopathic participants enumerated mostly events with the use of violence. In other words, the results can be considered from the point of view of aetiology and the development of psychopathic disorders. Thus, the theory of the deficit of basic emotional bonds brings attention to the fact that one of the most popular statements concerning the genesis of psychopathy, links its occurrence to an inappropriate family system in which a child lives during early childhood (Blackburn, 2003; Lykken, 2003; Pastwa-Wojciechowska, 2004; Farrington, 2007). It is assumed that from the moment of birth a child observes and then imitates the behaviour of its surroundings. In analysing the type of traumatic events enumerated by the participants, irregularities were observed, concerning both the family structure and relations within it. Interestingly, in a retrospective evaluation, one woman (mother, carer) was the weak person, submissive or reconciled to the aggression and violence of her husband (partner). She was so weak that she could not even develop her own status in the family, and the family relations put her into a position of failure to cope with life and the expectations of the family.

Considering the sex of participants, there were statistically significant differences between the male and female participants with regard to the experience of traumatic events, both in terms of their frequency and type. Only women experienced such events as sexual abuse in childhood, seeing another person with physical injuries or stealing without the use of violence, and they encountered more often events connected with the use of violence towards them or relatives. The results confirm the data found in the literature on the subject (Hare, 1970; Moretti et al., 1994; Beisert, 2004, Pastwa-Wojciechowska, 2004; Mac, 2005) stating that women, as being weaker, more often become the objects of aggressive behaviour and the witness of such events. As it turns out, in the case of women, even the factor of her height and strength is not enough to stop an offender from using violence. Even as an adult, the woman is still physically weaker and usually smaller than the man. Moreover, apart from physical or sexual violence, very often psychological violence was used towards women, which greatly influenced their mental and somatic condition. In other words, we can say that women were victims in their families, and they too would assume such a role as being the victim. Therefore, they adapted to the situation of being harmed (Pospiszyl, 2005). Men, on the other hand, experienced a real danger to their health and life, but they also pursued aggressive behaviour assuming a masculine pattern of behaviour, and thus they became offenders themselves.

Analysing the type and frequency of experienced traumatic events made it possible to determine the type of victimisation among the participants. It was found that the women most often experienced revictimisation with repeated victimisation. In other words, the acts of harm towards women were repeated and the offenders were either family members or other people. The men, on the other hand, experienced repeated victimisation, which means that the harm was mostly done by the same offender(s). It can be seen that both men and women experienced acts of harm by one or more offenders. However, the women were also harmed by other offenders more often. It can be concluded that a woman assuming the role of a victim resulted in her being perceived as weaker, which made it acceptable to use violence towards her (chronic victims) (Pospiszyl, 2003).

The last issue undertaken in this paper concerned the relation between the structure of psychopathy and type and frequency of experienced traumatic events. The results show that there is a relationship between the traits of psychopathic personality, perceived as important for the clinical diagnosis of psychopathic personality disorders, and such events as physical injury, a threat of using a firearm, physical abuse in childhood, seeing another person with physical injuries, stealing with the use of violence, attempted theft with the use of violence, and stealing without the use of violence. Interpreting the results we can say that there is a relationship between the experience of a traumatic event of a violent type and the development and shaping of a psychopathic personality. In other words, the results confirm the literature data concerning the existence of a relationship between physical harm and development of psychopathy (Raine, Sanmartin, 2001).

Recapitulating, people with a psychopathic personality structure often experienced harm in the form of physical violence in early childhood. It should be noted, however, that the women experienced harm from parents more often than the men. In other words, the women were perceived more often as weak and also assumed the role of victims themselves (being weak and allowing others to harm them) in the family. The men, on the other hand, more often became violent offenders towards other people themselves.

PART IV

NEUROBIOLOGICAL DISORDERS

CHAPTER NINE

POSTTRAUMATIC STRESS DISORDER FROM NEUROPHYSIOLOGY TO PSYCHOTHERAPY: A CROATIAN EXPERIENCE

RUDOLF GREGUREK

Introduction

War situations present individuals with probably the greatest quantity of most disturbing events succeeding one another or even coming together, creating extremely high pressure on all psychological defense models. War-related traumas include stressors of various natures, intensity, and duration, such as witnessing the death or wounding of a fellow soldier and/or civilians, being exposed to a sudden artillery and/or military attack, displacement, captivity, rape, and torture. Traumatic events may also be recurrent (Loncar, 2006).

During the 1991-1995 war in Croatia more than one million people were exposed to direct war stress. More than 13,000 individuals lost their lives, and over 33,000 were wounded. Among the wounded, more than 9,000 (9,816) were civilians. More than 1,000 (1,149) persons are still missing. The occupied areas of Croatia amounted to almost 15,000 square kilometers, or 26.5% of the state territory. Thus in these areas there were 549,083 inhabitants or 11.5% of the total population of Croatia (Hodalic, 1999; Torinek, 2005; Hebrang, 2006). Even more people were secondarily or vicariously traumatized. (Terzic, 2001; Vukusic, 2003). For instance, wives of the Croatian War veterans with PTSD suffered increased psychiatric symptoms, somatic complaints, and loneliness (Hebrang, et. al., 2006).

At the beginning of the 90's, knowledge about PTSD in Croatia was pretty poor and medical textbooks of psychiatry had only a few lines about that particular diagnostical entity. Therapeutic work, as well as the direct experience of a relationship with a patient who had PTSD, motivated us to try to define our own therapeutic approach that we based on our experience or possibilities (one could say education). One particular motive was the fact that society stigmatized this kind of patients.

The essential feature of posttraumatic stress disorder (PTSD) is the development of characteristic symptoms commonly divided into three symptom-clusters: persistent re-experiencing symptoms, avoidance and numbing symptoms and increased arousal (hyperarousal) symptoms (Yehuda, Davidson, 2002; Maes, et. al., 2000; Frommberger, 1998). The hyperarousal symptoms and persistent re-experiencing of the traumatic event suggest abnormalities in emotion and memory regulation, thus implicating limbic brain regions as possibly associated with the disorder. Recent brain neuroimaging studies have described several brain regions as possibly associated with PTSD symptoms. The most commonly described regions are limbic brain structures, the prefrontal cortex, and the temporal cortex (Liberzon, et. al., 1999; Bremner, 2000; Mirzaei, et. al., 2001; Pissota, et. al., 2002).

Our clinical experience has shown that hyperarousal symptoms present one of the dominant disturbances for chronic PTSD patients, especially those associated with impulsive aggressiveness such as hyperirritability, hyper excitability, hypersensitivity, aggressive acting-outs, and outbursts of anger. The elevated - arousal - state is likely to precipitate flight-or-fight reactions in these patients, so they often go immediately from stimulus to response without psychologically assessing the meaning of the event. This makes them prone to freeze or, alternatively, to overreact in response to minor provocations (van der Kolk, et. al., 1999).

The aim of our study was to assess possible changes in brain activation in PTSD patients after two years of intensive psychotherapy in the form of closed-door group analysis in a heterogeneous group specially designed in our clinic for treatment of PTSD patients.

Method

Participants in our study were selected from all PTSD patients treated at the Clinic for Psychological Medicine, University of Zagreb Medical School, in the period from April to July 2001. We selected 25 participants from a total of 82 patients treated in the day-hospital unit at the clinic over the period. All the participants in the study, as was most of our patients, were Croatian War (1991-1995) veterans who actively participated in combat and were exposed to multiple traumatic experiences such as witnessing the deaths of fellow soldiers and sudden air-rides or artillery attacks. (Patients who experienced other kinds of traumatic experiences such as being prisoners of war, concentration camp detainees, refugees, etc. were not included in this study.) They all signed informed consents to participate in the study.

Due to the high financial costs of the investigation procedure, participants were carefully selected on the basis of a specially designed inclusion procedure. The inclusion procedure consisted of a group evaluation and an individual psychiatric evaluation.

The group evaluation was performed over a two-week group psychotherapy period, as described above, encompassing four group sessions, and which consisted of monitoring the patients' symptom manifestations. The same co-therapist couple performed the selection for all the participants in the study. Individual evaluation was organized in the form of the Structured Clinical Interview for DSM-IV (SCID-CV) (First, 1996). The interview was held during the first week of the patients' treatment at the clinic, and was conducted by the same therapist for all participants. All therapists conducting the selection were clinicians with at last three years experience in working with psychotraumatized patients. Group therapists were not informed of the evaluation performed by the individual therapist, and conversely.

All patients selected for the investigation had chronic, combat-related PTSD with severe hyperarousal symptoms and impulsive aggressiveness and no other Axis-I and/or Axis-II diagnosis except for what was in accordance with the DSM-IV criteria (American Psychiatric Association, 1994). Severity of hyperarousal symptoms was assessed on the basis of anamnesis and heteroanamnesis and also on the basis of symptoms they manifested in group therapy and the individual psychiatric interview. Only those patients who continuously, over the two-week observation, presented all hyperarousal symptoms as defined in DSM-IV and showed impulsive aggressiveness symptoms were selected for the study. Impulsive aggressiveness symptoms were defined as hyperirritability, aggressive acting-outs, and outbursts of anger. Only patients who manifested these symptoms in both individual interviews and all four group sessions over the observation period, and who had positive anamnesis and heteroanamnesis for hyperarousal symptoms in the month preceding the hospitalization were included in the study. This selection design had to be implemented because no psychometric instrument for assessing hyperarousal and/or impulsive aggressiveness symptoms as such, qualitatively or preferably quantitatively, was available in Croatia.

The patients selected for the study received nothing other than benzodiazepine pharmacotherapy for at least six months preceding the study, and four weeks before the study entry, patients received no psychotropic medication at all. After the psychiatric evaluation, a neurological examination was conducted for all participants to exclude those with possible neurological comorbid conditions, head trauma or loss of consciousness in the year preceding the study.

All patients included in the study were male, right-handed, of similar age (mean=42 years, SD=2), and had no history of alcohol or drug abuse or dependence.

Single Photon Emission Computed Tomography (SPECT) using Tc^{99}-ECD functional brain imaging was organized in the week after the two-week observation period immediately after the first group session in that week to establish possible alterations in regional cerebral blood flow (rCBF). The procedure was organized in the following way. Patients who manifested at least one and no more than three aggressive acting-outs during the pre-SPECT session were asked to remember the specific situation in the group that provoked the last aggressive acting-out. The ultimate of no more than three aggressive acting-outs during the designated session was a pre-set criteria to enable remembering of the specific situation that provoked the last acting-out, but was not used since none of our subjects actually manifested more than three aggressive acting-outs during the pre-SPECT session. The subjects were asked to try to remember the exact situation in the group that provoked their aggressive acting-out and to describe it. Only the subjects who were able to do this and who manifested aggression and anger while remembering, and also who felt distressed by that were included in the further procedure. Once again all of our subjects fulfilled these criteria and all were declared very distressed when remembering the situation. Following this, subjects were introduced into the SPECT procedure, and scans were obtained in 50 to 60 minutes after the end of the session. Once again immediately before the SPECT brain scan was made, each subject was asked to remember the situation that provoked his last aggressive acting-out in the pre-SPECT session.

SPECT scans were started 20 minutes after the administration of 740 MBq of 99mTc-ECD in a resting state ("white noise" environment, without any auditory or visual combat stimuli provocation). Measurements were made with an IRIX triple-headed rotating scintillation gamma camera fitted with high-resolution collimators, using a 360° circular orbit and step and shoot mode (20-s image each 3°) , each acquisition lasting 40 minutes. Within-subject correlated slices were obtained. Images were acquired in a 128x128 matrix, with an acquisition zoom of 1.5. The final pixel size was 2.96 mm. The full-width at half-maximum (FWHM) in the transaxial plane was 9 mm. Filtered back-projection was used for reconstruction by applying a Metz filter. Attenuation correction of the reconstructed data was applied using Chang's method, with a coefficient factor of 0.075. Two-pixel-thick slices were obtained in the coronal, sagittal and oblique (fronto-occipital) planes.

SPECT data were quantitatively analyzed using an Odyssey FX820 workstation by means of a region-of-interest (ROI) based method and calculation of asymmetry percentages. The following ROIs were considered: temporal, frontal, orbitofrontal and occipital cortices, cingulate gyrus, amygdala, thalamus, basal ganglia (caudate, putamen, ventral basal ganglia) and cerebellum. The irregular ROIs were outlined in the right hemisphere and mirrored in the left. The same investigator, blinded for all clinical data, placed the ROIs. For each ROI, mean counts per pixel in two consecutive slices were averaged to minimize partial volume effects. In each patient, studies were normalized to the mean whole-brain uptake; so relative hypo/hyperperfusion was established for each ROI. The percentage of asymmetry between two homologous regions was calculated as 200x (right-left/right+left), where right and left indicate mean average counts per pixel in the ROIs of the respective hemisphere. Thus the negative values indicate lower perfusion in the right hemisphere. Percentages of interhemispheric asymmetry between homologous brain regions were used to identify abnormalities.

Therapy

Patients were subdued to a group psychotherapy used in the form of wclosed-door group analysis with a once-a week 90-minute session rate, focusing on patients' interpersonal and social relations and communication, specially designed in our clinic for treatment of PTSD patients. The group had 10 members: six men (Croatian war veterans) and four women (partners of the war veterans, who were not related to the men in the group). During the psychotherapy period the patient consumed no pharmacotherapy, except anxiolytic (benzodiazepine) therapy over the first three weeks of the therapy in order to alleviate acute symptoms and enable the psychotherapeutic process.

People whose reactions to early traumas have become integrated into the totality of their personalities are apt to repeat aspects of the trauma and defensive reactions to trauma in their relationships with other people. In heterogeneous, transference-oriented trauma groups, the social expressions of those trauma-related affects and cognitive schemata are inevitably expressed on a social level and became readily observable.

Long-term heterogeneous groups can be particularly helpful to people with previous individual therapy, where they have an opportunity to develop a language in which they can identify their feelings and a basic curiosity about how they themselves may contribute to solve their problems in interpersonal relationships. Patients "fitting" for the group analysis should have the ability to observe their own problems, the ability to react emotionally, as well as have a certain capacity to save somebody else's emotions and the capacity for insight (Gregurek, 1999).

The therapeutic environment should be created in a way that enables individuals who are similar in some way to understand and feel with others, but at the same time different enough so they can watch and help other group members from different perspectives and positions. The best group composition is when the members are similar in terms of ego-development and different in terms of interpersonal style. Groups which are focused on the relationships between their members allow new losses to be experienced, as object loses with concomitant grief and sadness, rather than with narcissistic injuries accompanied by feelings of helplessness, numbing, and vengeful rage. As heterogeneous trauma groups mature, they gradually make that transition. When that happens, the group members start getting the full benefit of the strengths that traumatized persons have developed to survive catastrophic trauma.

Results

Based on studies of normal subjects, it is well documented that normal cerebral blood distribution is bilaterally symmetric, with percentages of interhemispheric asymmetry never exceeding 12% for any brain region (Juni, et. al., 1998; Koyama, et. al., 1997; Camarago, 2004). In our study the SPECT brain scans, at the beginning of the psychotherapeutic treatment, with a two-week period between, showed a unilateral (dominant brain hemisphere) 20% or more increase in the regional blood flow (rCBF) in the projection area of the ventral basal ganglia (VBG) (Image 4-1). Also, due to the well-documented normal brain perfusion patterns in the SPECT study - paralleling our own 10-year experience - and due to the radioactive properties of the method coupled with high financial costs of the procedure, it was ethically and financially impossible for us to include a control group of normal subjects.

After two years of group psychotherapy, PTSD patients' symptoms diminished and they regained adequate impulse control. Control SPECT scans were performed on two separate occasions with a three-week period in-between. No differences from the normal pattern were found (Image4-2).

Discussion

We found unilaterally increased perfusion in the projection area of the ventral basal ganglia (VBG) in the dominant brain hemisphere, in our PTSD subjects with severe hyperarousal symptoms and impulsive aggressiveness, and after two years of group psychotherapy our patients show no differences from their normal pattern. One possible conclusion is that SPECT findings are associated with the symptoms of PTSD. They receded together with the clinical manifestation of symptoms; so it could be used as a neurobiological indicator in order to make a psychotherapeutical intervention focused on symptoms and clinical remission yet neurobiologically verified, as in our study. Symptoms of arousal, especially symptoms of increased impulsive aggression in an ethiopathological sense, are exaggerated; and the adaptive inadequate reactivity of the psychical apparatus on emotional triggers from the environment or inner psychical world of the sufferer [equally specific ones] - are trauma-related and non-specifically usual for human experience in general.

Over-aggressive reacting to normally meek emotional stimuli as a lack of impulse control symptoms, can in that respect be understood as an over-defensive, mal-adaptive response. It is convincible to believe that SPECT findings as described above are associated with the lack of impulse control symptoms (Liberzon, et. al., 1999).

Response to stress results in a multitude of biological and psychological changes designed to prepare the body for fight-or-flight situations. As part of the stress response, a cascade of biochemical changes occur in the hypothalamus, pituitary, and adrenal glands (the HPA axis), as well as in the sympathetic nervous system. These biochemical changes mediate the physical and psychological changes experienced during stress and crisis.

Trauma is biochemically encoded in the brain in a variety of ways, including changes in the availability and effects of neurotransmitters and neuromodulators. Neuroanatomic encoding occurs through changes in structures like the hippocampus, through coordination and integration of the neural network functioning.

The hyperarousal symptoms and persistent re-experiencing of the traumatic event suggest abnormalities in emotion and memory regulation, thus implicating limbic brain regions as possibly associated with the disorder.

VBG, which corresponds to the anatomical location of the Nucleus accumbens, is functionally and spatially closely related to the amygdala (Lang, et. al., 1998; Davis, Whalen, 2001; Zahm, 1999; LeDoux, 1986). Both structures together have been implicated in adaptive responding and non-declarative emotional memory (Lang, et. al., 1998; Davis, Whalen, 2001; Zahm, 1999; LeDoux, 1986; Yehuda, Davidson, 2002). Adaptive responding is a process by which an organism, having extracted information from its external environment and internal milieu, interprets and utilizes those cues in creating an appropriate emotional response to incoming stimuli. Nucleus accumbens receives inputs primarily from the highest order of the integrative, polymodal cortical and cortical-like structures, such as the prefrontal cortex, basal amygdala and subiculum. It also projects mainly to the basal forebrain, dienchephalon and rostral brainstem. In this way the nucleus accumbens appears to be a sensitive recipient of information about the hedonic/ aversive valences of incoming stimuli and appropriately stimulates or inhibits activity in brain structures with more direct capacities to affect the decision-making, initiation and motor control aspects of adaptive responding. The way it fashions these functions is nevertheless still largely vague.

Hyperarousal symptoms within PTSD can, at least to some extent, be explained by malfunction of the Nucleus accumbens and related limbic brain structures and the psychological processes they mediate (Yehuda, Davidson, 2002; van der Kolk, et. al., 1999; Zubieta, et. al., 1999; Bremner, et. al., 1993; LeDoux, 1986). Hyperirritability, hyperexcitability, hypersensitivity in this respect that they present inadequate, exaggerated responses ("emergency" fight-or-flight reactions) to information that would normally produce a reaction of a considerably modest extent, can be associated with the malfunction of the adaptive responding process.

That is why we believe that the increased rCBF in the projection area of the Nucleus accumbens found in our subjects might substantiate for any disturbed neuronal activity in this region, thus allowing for the disturbances in the psychological processes it mediates. Unfortunately, it was impossible for us to quantitatively measure hyperarousal symptoms and/or impulsive aggressiveness in our subjects, and to correlate these with the alterations in rCBF. This was due to the lack of adequate psychometric instruments in Croatia. Perhaps subjects with changed rCBF patterns had more severe symptoms in this respect. Due to reasons mentioned above it was also not possible for us to more specifically define and quantify the symptom profile in each subject regarding different hyperarousal / impulsive aggressiveness symptoms. We believe this would possibly yield some additional information and explain normal findings in almost half of our subjects.

Changes in neurobiological mechanisms are reflected in the victim's psychological, physiological, and interpersonal experiences. A deficit in psychological and interpersonal functioning then creates additional stress, which further compromises neurobiological structures. This way, adaptation to trauma, especially early in life, becomes a "state of mind, brain, and body" around which all subsequent experiences are organized (Gold, 2005).

Treatment goals of psychodynamic approaches to PTSD are to restore normal intrapsychic functioning. Psychodynamic approaches to the treatment of PTSD place emphasis on levels of conscious awareness of dysregulated psychobiological processes.

From the perspective of neuroscience, psychotherapy can be understood as a specific kind of enriched environment designed to enhance the growth of neurons and the integration of neural networks (Corrigan, 2004; Fuchs, 2004). The therapeutic environment is individually tailored to fit the symptoms and needs of the patient. On the neurological level, this equates to the integration and communication of neural networks dedicated to emotion, cognition, sensation, and behavior. On a psychological level, integration is the ability to experience the important aspects of life while employing a minimum of defenses. Growth and integration are optimized by a positive early environment, including stage-appropriate challenges, support, and parents who are capable and willing to put feelings into words (Kandel, 1999).

These factors lead to positive affect regulation, biological homeostasis, and a quiet "internal milieu" allowing for the consolidation of the experience of subjectivity and a positive sense of self.

It is possible to conclude that SPECT findings are associated with the symptoms of PTSD. They receded together with the clinical manifestation of symptoms; so it could be used as a neurobiological indicator in order to make a psychotherapeutical intervention which is focused on symptoms and clinical remission but which can be neurobiologically verified, as in the Seedat (2004) study. Functional brain imaging has opened a window to the living human brain in the acts of motor tasks, in experiencing symptoms, imagining a feared situation, or in telling a lie. An examination of areas activated during different tasks has enhanced our understanding of which neural networks participate in various functions.

As scanning techniques become more precise and the hardware more affordable, they will without doubt become incorporated into the treatment of

PTSD and other disorders. As part of the initial assessment, they could help therapists pinpoint areas of neural activation and inhibition. Treatment planning will come to include specific psychotherapeutic and pharmacological intervention to enhance the growth and integration of affected networks.

Regular scans during the course of therapy may someday replace psychological tests as ways of fine-tuning the therapeutic process and measuring treatment success. The psychiatrist himself must think about the whole person first, and appreciate that each one is interesting and unique, not simply a composite of symptoms that are used to make an ICD or DSM diagnosis and provide treatment according to a standard algorithm.

Figure 9-1 SPECT brain scans at the beginning of psychotherapeutic treatment, with a two-week period between

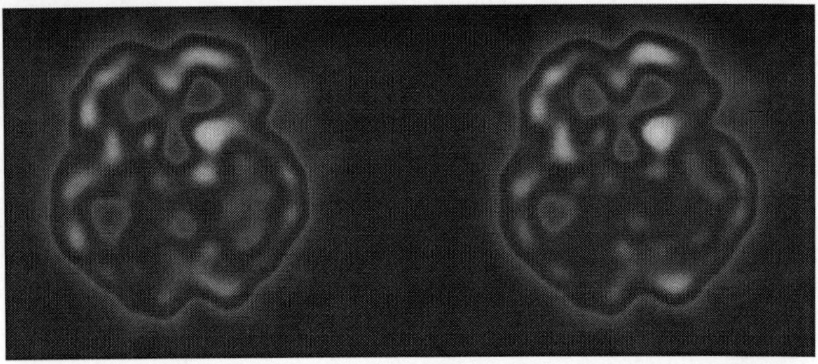

Figure 9-2 SPECT brain scans at the end of the psychotherapeutic treatment, with three-week period between

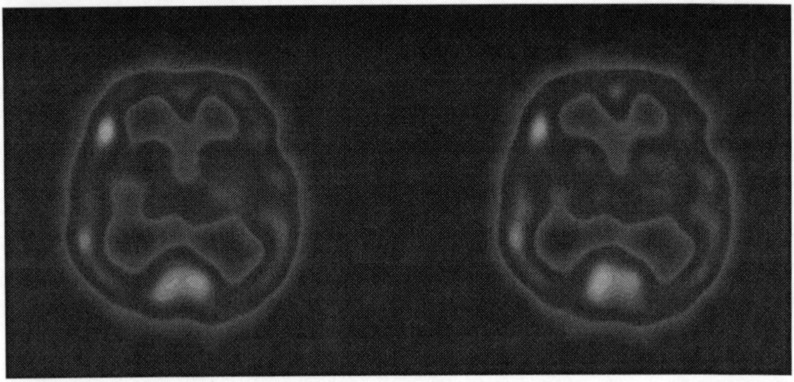

CHAPTER TEN

CHANGES IN SENSING, THE BASIC FUNCTION OF BODY EGO, AS A RESULT OF TRAUMA

OLGA SAKSON-OBADA

Abnormalities within body experience are considered one of the consequences of trauma (Cole and Putnam, 1992; Herman, 2003; van der Kolk, 2003). They involve such diverse phenomena as a negative attitude toward one's own body (Andrews, 1995; Harned, 2000), dissociation from the body (Nijenhuis et al., 1998), or lack of the ability to protect one's own body (Wycisk, 2004).In describing different aspects of body experience influenced by trauma, authors do not draw any consistent classification of disturbances, and do not put them into basic personality constructs. The question arises as to whether various aspects of body experience changed by trauma can be organized within the framework of a theoretical construct such as body ego or body self.

Although in recent years we have been observing a growing interest in the problem of body self and body ego [1] in the context of the psychological functioning of a human being (Kowalik, 2003; Kruger, 2002; Mirucka, 2003; Sakson-Obada, 2009; Schier, 2009) we also observe the a lack of common understanding of these aspects of personality. An analysis of literature allows one to postulate that though there is common agreement that body ego and body self are related to the way one experiences his or her body, firstly, there is still no consistent idea what this notion actually means and, secondly, it is still not clear what kinds of corporeality are crucial for the psychological functioning of a human being.

The notion of body ego-an attempt at defining it

When confronting the lack of a consistent model of body ego (and body self), it is worthwhile starting from an attempt at defining this notion, before presenting the hypotheses and results of studies on disturbances within one of the functions of body ego, namely sensing stimuli coming both from the environment and the interior of one's body.

Consequently, I assumed that body ego is a part of ego structure, a part which organizes the body experiences in the form of representations whose quality determines the way a person experiences oneself, that is, experiences his or her sense of physical identity. Thus body ego is a subsystem of ego, since unlike psychological ego it is responsible for processing bodily experience on the mental plane. In the proposed view, body ego is the instance that integrates bodily experience (compare the concept of body *ego* - Anzieu, 1979; Hoffer, 1950; Szasz, 1957), in the form of representations (compare the concept of body *self* - Krueger, 2002; Mahler and McDevitt, 1982) on the basis of which the sense of physical identity is built. In the view proposed here body ego is an autonomous instance of personality and it is identical with the notion of the executive aspect of *Ich* (ie. *ego*), defined within the framework of psychodynamic theories (conf. Laplanche, Pontalis, 1996, p. 100).

Organising bodily experiences is possible due to particular functions of body ego, acquired in the course of development, and presented in the model below:

Figure 10-1 Model of body ego

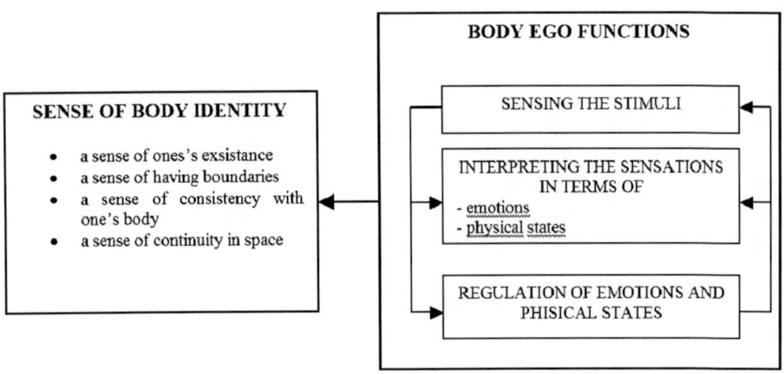

The first function of body ego is sensing the stimuli coming both from the environment and from the interior of the body. The second function of body ego is interpreting the sensations such as emotions and physical states (eg. hunger, tiredness or sexual arousal). The third of the distinguishing functions is regulation of emotions and physical states, thus recognizing the reasons for, and ways to cope, with emotions and physical states. The capability to operate with the above functions, acquired and mastered in the process of development, makes it possible for the bodily identity to find its support in increasingly differentiated and internally integrated representations of the sensations coming from the environment and from the body itself. In the case of a healthy, adult person such aspects of a sense of bodily identity as (a) a sense of one's own existence, (b) a sense of having boundaries, (c) a sense of consistency with one's own body, (d) and its continuity in space, are not consciously perceived (verbalized) in the categories of any aspect of the *self*. Many authors assume that the normal relationship between body and mind entails "the state of quiet cooperation", where bodily functioning does not preoccupy the attention of an individual excessively (Erikson, 1956; Torras de Bea, 1987). In this respect, the sense of one's own identity (bodily identity) most frequently remains a "silent" experience, mainly due to the ability of body ego to smoothly integrate the experiences constituting it.

In the model presented here, sensing stimuli, both external, and internal ones, is considered a basic function to the effect that it is a condition without which it would be useless to talk about the other functions. In other words, the inability to perceive stimuli coming from the environment or from the interior of one's own body significantly impairs or even frustrates recognizing and controlling one's own bodily experience, either in the form of emotions or physical states. It is impossible for me to recognize my own bodily state as fear or sexual arousal if I do not feel the changes occurring in my own body. At this point it is worth noting that abnormalities within one of the functions of body ego, such as sensing, may manifest themselves as a decrease or an increase in sensitivity to stimuli. The latter type of abnormality would be observed when, for example, subtle touch is experienced as painful, or when minor changes in the operation of internal organs is perceived as intense.

Sensing stimuli and trauma

Attempting to explain the disturbances within sensing, one finds in literature devoted to the problem of traumas mainly clinical reports presenting decreased sensitivity to external stimuli (Herman, 2003; van der Kolk et al,. 1985; van der Kolk and Saporta, 1993; Terr, 1991). Most authors focus their attention on blunted sensing of pain or touch stimuli, accompanying not only the state of dissociation but also viewed as a permanent characteristic of individuals who experienced chronic suffering in their past. The defensive character of this abnormality may be expressed as follows: *I stop to feel in order not to suffer*. However, studies on somatomorphic dissociation showed as well that victims of trauma replied affirmatively when asked questions concerning excessive sensitivity to touch, sound or visual stimuli (Nijenhuis et al., 1998).

Considering this information, it seemed interesting to investigate whether in victims of trauma, the episodes of disturbance in sensing are unidirectional, consisting in either an increase or decrease of sensory thresholds or in the possibility that they co-ocur.

Although researchers of the consequences of trauma do not discuss the problem of sensing stimuli coming from the interior of the body, it seems that the assumptions made by authors dealing with the phenomenon of interoception (Schmidt, Lerew and Trakowski, 1997; Cameron, 2001; Mussgay, Klinkenberg and Ruddel, 1999) substantiate posing an interesting research problem concerning the changes in this sphere of body ego in victims of trauma. These authors take the view that a decreased ability to perceive stimuli from the interior of the body is related to the defensive avoidance of stimuli, whenever their frequency and/or intensity is a source of intolerable distress. It may thus be expected that chronic trauma may lead to decreased sensitivity to internal bodily stimuli.

It is worth mentioning, though, that there exist data pointing to a link between increased awareness of sensations the source of which is one's own body, with the number of adverse events that took place in the course of the life of an individual (Baradell and Klein, 1993). A question then arises whether increased sensitivity to sensation coming from the interior of the body may also be an effect of trauma.

To summarize the above discussion, it may be assumed as probable that in some individuals a traumatic experience may lead to increased sensitivity to stimuli coming from the interior of their bodies, while in others it may lead to defensive evasion of the same stimuli.

Based on the presented studies, clinical reports and theoretical assumptions, it was expected that the greater the intensity of trauma, the more likely it is that the following disturbances within body ego will occur: lifting or lowering the pain or touch threshold (for experiencing the external stimuli), and a greater or smaller less than average number of registered sensations coming from the body (for experiencing stimuli coming from the body), accompanied by inadequate appraisal of one's own arousal.

In the study, the following variables were tested

1. touch threshold
2. pain threshold
3. In the category of sensing stimuli coming from the body, two variables were considered:
   a. the number of sensations coming from the body;
   b. a subjective appraisal of the intensity of arousal

Each of these variables was tested separately in the course of the procedure of hyperventilation and interpersonal touch.

Trauma was considered the independent variable. Its intensity was determined by the particular kinds of trauma experienced as well as by the circumstances accompanying it.

Method

Subjects and course of study

The subjects of research have been selected during screening conducted from May 2005 to September 2006 among students of three higher education colleges in Poznań, Poland. The aim of the screening was to select a group that would enter the research proper on the basis of the results of the self-report pertaining to the body ego. Because of the major goal of the research (verification of the model of body ego), the procedure of the screening had been planned so as to select 50 subjects with the highest and 50 subjects with the lowest results in the questionnaire from a total of 200 participants. In order to obtain 200 for this further part of the study, it was necessary to examine 938 persons (393 males and 545 females). In the final research 105 subjects were engaged (28 males and 77 females), aged 19 to 30 ($M = 21,8$; $SD = 2,61$).

The research proper involved individual sessions with a trained experimenter, during which the subjects filled in a questionnaire and participated in the procedures, serving the purpose of the major project. Individual meetings lasted from 50 minutes to one and a half hours. The methods used for verification of the hypotheses presented here will be described below.

Instruments and procedures

A Temp Test device for examining the pain thresholds. This apparatus was constructed for the purpose of this study by a company named EIEWIN, following a design described in psychological literature of a device meant for examining sensitivity to pain, the pain being induced by warming a part of an individual's body (conf. Orbach et al., 1997). The device comprises a heating element, a setting mechanism for controlling the operation of the apparatus, communication with a computer, and a manipulator (a key on the computer keyboard) enabling the subject to signal. After the subject put his hand on the heating element, the following instruction was given: "*In a while the temperature will stabilize at thirty degrees (Celsius). After ten seconds I will inform you that the device has begun to operate, and then you will feel that the temperature will slowly grow. As soon as you feel burning pain, Press ENTER on the black keyboard and remove your hand from the plate*".

The subjects placed the palm of their hands on the heating element, an aluminium plate 55mm x 25mm in such a way that the whole surface of their hands was touching the heating area. Ten seconds after the subject placed hand on the plate, the experimenter turned on heating, and informed the subject about it. The device was turned off when the subject pressed the key of the manipulator held in his or her hand. Three measures were taken at three-minute intervals (conf. Orbach, Mikulincer and King, 1997). For calculation purposes the mean value of the three rates was computed.

Semmes-Weinstein Estesiometer. The device serves to estimate sensitivity to touch as pressure. It is built of twenty nylon fibres embedded at an acute angle in plastic handles. For each fibre a minimal strength of pressure necessary to bend it is defined (from 0.0045 g to 448 g). Considering the data on the relationship between care and sensitivity to touch in the right hand fingers (Kozłowska 1998), it was decided that this part of skin will be examined. Estimation of the touch threshold consisted in finding the thinnest fibre whose pressure the subject could perceive.

Hyperventilation and interpersonal touch procedures. This test served to estimate the number of bodily sensations registered by the subjects of the study. In order to induce arousal, two independent procedures were used: hyperventilation and interpersonal touch procedures. It started with introducing the subjects to the following instructions:

Instruction for hyperventilation

The task will consist of six deep inhalations and exhalations: Please breathe at the following rate: (The experimenter demonstratd the pace of breathing-one cycle took three seconds).

Instruction for touch

Now I am going to put my hand on your forearm, and we will stay this way for a while (the experimenter held her hand for eight seconds).

After the hyperventilation and touch ceased, the subjects were asked to focus on their experience, and reply to the question: *What was going on in your body?* in order to report the perceived changes. Their replies were registered on a special spreadsheet prepared for the purpose of the study.

Traumatic Experiences Questionnaire. The instrument served to assess the presence of traumatic experiences and their circumstances, and was developed for the purpose of this study, whose part is the subject of this paper. The questionnaire comprises 22 statements describing emotionally burdening events related to experiencing one of five types of trauma. Thus the measure consists of five subscales: (1) physical abuse (Cronbach's α = 0. 71; e.g.: "I was beaten and I did not know what for"), (2) sexual abuse (Cronbach's $\alpha = 0.61$; e.g. "I was forced into having sex against my will"), (3) emotional neglect (Cronbach's $\alpha = 0.78$; e.g. "I felt they wouldn't care if I died"), (4) emotional abuse (Cronbach's $\alpha = 0.73$; "When I wanted to cuddle up, I was pushed away or told to go away"), (5) physical neglect (Cronbach's $\alpha = 0.37$; e.g.: "Nobody cared if I had anything to eat"[2]), and (6) witnessing trauma. The additional questions were added about experiencing (7) divorce or separation of parents, (8) separation with a loved one, (9) death of a loved one, (10) a serious car accident, and (11) intense physical pain. The measure of trauma was a simple sum total of all traumatic experiences. Apart from a simple summing up of responses to particular questions referring to the described category, the questionnaire encompassed also those circumstances of the traumatic event that, based on literature, were likely to increase the risk of developing disorders. These were age at which an event was experienced (refers to all variables), frequency of the event, person responsible for the event, and number of the persons responsible (variables 1-6); intensity of sense of helplessness and terror (variables 1-9), objective stimulus' impact (variables 10-11). Additionally, another variable was distinguished, namely the intensity of the trauma, reflected in the sum total of all traumatic experiences, with consideration of all the additional points for accompanying circumstances.[3]

Results

The gathered data was subject to statistical analysis (with the use of the package SPSS. 12.0.). In order to verify the hypothesis on the relationship of trauma with lifted and lowered touch thresholds, one-variable variance analysis was used. Using this method, in which three groups of women were studied [4] and who were assigned to the groups based on the level of pain and touch thresholds they revealed, no significant differences between these groups were found with respect to the intensity of traumatic experiences, and the total trauma impact,. In order to reply to the question, whether any kind of dependency exists between the pain and touch thresholds, and trauma, a correlation method was used. The analysis was conducted separately for groups of men and women, and its results are presented in the table below.

Table 10-1. Corelations different types of trauma with pain threshold and touch threshold

	Pain threshold		Touch threshold	
	Males	Females	Males	Females
Emotional abuse	.050	-.106	-.276	.070
Physical abuse	**-334**(*)	-.078	-.206	**.447**(**)
Sexual abuse	-.171	.074	-.045	.136
Physical neglect	.065	-.099	.111	-.035
Emotional neglect	-.036	**-.205**(*)	**-.339**(*)	.033
Witnessing trauma	.113	**-.224**(*)	-.299	.131
Divorce	.113	-.045	-.308	-.007
Separation with loved one	.020	-.052	**-.381**(*)	-.091
Death of love one	.129	.093	-.023	.073
Intensity of trauma	.004	**-.190**(*)	-.278	.149

*Note.***p* <.05. ***p* <.01

As it appears from the above data, in the group of women there is a relationship of pain threshold with two types of trauma, and the total trauma impact. The correlations are negative, meaning that in the group of woman emotional neglect and witnessing trauma, and the total sum of the trauma, are accompanied with excessive sensitivity to pain. As far as the variable touch threshold is concerned, we found a positive correlation between this variable and physical abuse. The result means that lifted touch threshold in the group of women was accompanied with experience of physical suffering inflicted by other people.

In the male group, the pain threshold correlated negatively with one type of trauma only. Excessive sensitivity to pain then was accompanied in men by the experience of physical violence. The touch threshold variable was accompanied with three types of trauma, and was negatively correlated with each of these types. The result means that lowered touch threshold was accompanied with emotional neglect, separation with a loved person, and experienced intense pain. The acquired data confirm expectations only partially. It had been assumed that not only excessive sensitivity to pain, but also blunted perception of it would be related to trauma (in the light of the acquired data, the second part of the hypothesis must be discarded). Analogous results were expected while investigating the relationships between touch thresholds and trauma. The acquired results, indeed, show that changes in touch thresholds caused by trauma may consist in either decreased or increased sensitivity to this type of stimuli, but the direction of these changes depends on gender.

Experiencing stimuli coming from the body and trauma

Another research question was whether the number of registered stimuli is related to traumatic experiences. It was expected that both a lack of, and excessive number of, registered bodily changes is related to trauma. In order to verify this hypothesis the intensity of particular traumatic experiences was compared in the groups of subjects who experienced various numbers of sensations during in the situation/touch and hyperventilation procedures. Single-variable variance analysis proved no statistically significant differences with respect to particular types of trauma or total intensity of trauma between the groups of people ascribed to different groups, based on various numbers of sensations registered in the situation of being touched. The result would suggest that there exists no relationship between the number of sensations experienced in the situation of being touched and trauma; however - as we would see further on - correlation analysis would question such a conclusion.

The results of variance analysis for groups of subjects differing in the number of sensations reported in the situation of hyperventilation proved there were significant differences with respect to two types of trauma - sexual abuse and death of a loved one - between persons differing with respect to the number of sensations reported in the situation of hyperventilation. Thus, as far as sexual abuse is concerned, a difference was found between persons reporting one or two sensations, and those who reported the maximum number of them (ie. four, $F(4.100) = 2.58$; $p =$ 0.42). In the case of the death of a beloved person, a difference was found between persons reporting feeling no bodily changes and those who reported the greatest number of such changes (F (4.100) = 3.40; p = 0.,12). The acquired data suggest that only two types of trauma are related to the number of sensations registered in situations of hyperventilation. Moreover, it is possible to conclude that the intensity of two types of trauma are greater only in the group of persons reporting the maximum number of sensations in the hyperventilation procedure, compared to people who did not admit to sensing any bodily changes or admitted to only two of such changes.

It was decided as well to check whether correlation analysis reveals any new information on the link between registered sensations and trauma. The results of this analysis are presented in the Table below.

Table 10-2. Corelations of different types of trauma with number of registered stimuli

	Number having sensation in hiperventilation	**Number having sensation in the touch procedure**
Emotional abuse	.148	.202(*)
Physical abuse	.076	.140
Sexual abuse	**.225(*)**	**.218(*)**
Physical neglect	.084	**.207(*)**
Emotional neglect	.154	**.237(**)**
Witnessing trauma	.077	.160
Divorce	.055	-.085
Separation with a loved one	.055	.048
Death of a love one	**.302(**)**	.030
Intensity of trauma	**.172(*)**	**.225(*)**
*Note.***p* <.05. ***p* <.01		

According to the data presented in the Table, the number of sensations reported in the situation of hyperventilation correlated positively with total trauma intensity and with two types of trauma only, namely with sexual abuse and death of a beloved person. Registering numerous bodily changes when being touched was accompanied with total trauma intensity, and such types of trauma as emotional abuse, sexual abuse, and physical and emotional neglect. The results do not confirm the part of the hypothesis that assumed co-ocurrence of trauma with a lack of registering changes in the body. Correlation analysis showed more links between particular types of trauma and the number of sensations registered in situation of being touched than in the situation of hyperventilation. It is worth remarking that depending on the type of experimental procedures (touch or hyperventilation) used, the discussed variable is linked with various types of trauma. This data would suggest that consequences of a particular type of trauma in the form of intensified registration of sensations coming from the body manifest themselves in particular circumstances; they are not of a trans-situational nature.

The results suggest that the relational context is of remarkable importance when awareness of sensations in individuals who experienced suffering inflicted by others is considered. Excessive reactions, consisting in registering a great number of changes, manifest themselves more clearly in response to touch initiated by the experimenter than to changes induced by hyperventilation. This kind of reaction seems to be an „alarm" signal for the victims of trauma, serving as information that helps to increase vigilance when physical closeness is associated with shaken security.

Summary

The presented results arrange themselves in a coherent picture whose leading leitmotiv is hypersensitivity both to external stimuli and to stimuli coming from the interior of the body. In my view it is an interesting result, considering the fact that in literature mainly blunting of sensitivity, particularly cutting-off from sensations is highlighted. Where, then, do such literature results come from, being - one could say - biased and inconsistent with observations of persons working with victims of trauma on a day-to-day basis? It is worth remembering that information on blunted pain sensation in victims of trauma were formulated based on data about their co-ocurrence with the states of dissociation. It is then possible that in a "normal" state of consciousness victims of trauma are hypersensitive to such stimuli as pain, touch or the stimuli taking its source in an individual's own body, which might be considered an adaptive prevention mechanism.

Another explanation may be the weight of a trauma. It is possible therefore that only the most severe traumas, continuing for many years, result in the individual's engaging a substantially more serious psychological defence mechanism, such as cutting-off from sensing the severe trauma. In the studied group, there were only few persons chronically experiencing abuse (physical and sexual); therefore it is possible that we would acquire a different view of the studied relationships if we examined persons who were exposed to prolonged abuse that had begun early in their childhood.

It is also possible that other variables modifying the consequences of experiencing trauma have not been discussed in the presented study (eg. anxiety as a state or attachment pattern).

Notes

[1] In Polish there is no distinction between the concepts of self, ego and I. All these terms are expressed with one word "I". This fact complicates translation. I assume that "ego" refers to the executive aspect of personality, and the self refers to representations.

[2] Low value of reliability suggest that experiences belonging to the category "physical abuse" do not have to co-occur. Although these experiences do not have any characteristics of a syndrome, it was decided to include data acquired from the application of this scale.

[3] Thus, apart from a simple summing up of affirmative answers to questions concerning particular traumatic events, additional points were granted when specific circumstances of trauma occurred and were considered as increasing the risk of disturbance. An additional point was granted for the following situations: (1) trauma took place when the subject was younger than six; (2) when it occurred several times in a month; (3) the abuser (or victim) was a person from the family of origin; (4) there were three or more abusers (or victims); (5) the sum total of replies concerning experience of fear and helplessness was six or more; (6) when the person was very much afraid about his or her health or was sure he or she would die when experiencing the disaster; (7) when he or she was seriously injured as a result of an accident; (8) experienced prolonged pain (no matter how intensive).

[4] The decision to discontinue conducting the analysis for the male group was dictated by the fact that there were not enough subjects to divide them into three groups (lowered, average, lifted thresholds) in a reasonable way.

PART V

PSYCHOLOGICAL TRAUMA TREATMENT

CHAPTER ELEVEN

DOMESTIC VIOLENCE INTERVENTION BY WELFARE WORKERS AND LAYPERSONS

ALICJA KUCZYŃSKA
AND ALICJA STRZELECKA-LEMIECH

The Word Health Organization defines violence as "the intentional use of force or power, threatened or actual, against oneself, another person or against a group or community, that either results in or has a high likelihood of resulting in injury, death, psychological harm, maldevelopment, or deprivation" (Word Health Organization Global Consultation on Violence & Health, 1996, p. 3-4). As evidenced by the results of considerable research, violence can also have less visible and long-term consequences. For example adverse childhood experiences increase risks later in life of heart disease, cancer, depression, suicide, substance abuse, unintended pregnancy and sexually transmitted disease (Briere, 1986; Wycisk, in this book). Intimate partner violence encourages the risk of developing asthma, arthritis, stroke, heavy or binge drinking (Campbell, 2002, for a review).

The widespread problem, and complex individual and social consequences, of violence tend to make all efforts aim at preventing and reducing all its forms. The most planned, organized and systematic efforts in this direction are taken by public institutions (Hammond, et al, 2009), which are often supported by social organizations. Scientists also participate substantially in these activities ; they try to describe the problem, recognize its causes and consequences, develop strategies to help solve it, and indicate the factors which prevent the rise of the problem. However, the efforts and activities of public organizations and scientists are not able to replace the importance of direct response people being the witness of violence. Proceeding from this assumption we conducted research aimed at testing the influence of collateral factors pertaining to violence that is on helping social workers and non-professional persons to intervene in such circumstances.

Domestic violence in Poland

A precise evaluation of domestic violence is very difficult and depends on who, when, from whom and in what way data is collected that will serve as the basis for the evaluation. For instance police and welfare services usually register only the reported cases of domestic violence, and in Poland police data does not include cases where victims have withdrawn their complaint (Nowakowska, Jabłońska, 1998).

Results of polls and interviews depend not only on the size and level of sample representativeness , but also on characteristics and behaviors of the interviewers and those who give the data (for instance their consent or refusal to participate in the interview, willingness to tell the truth or conceal their experiences (Crowne and Marlowe, 1964, as cited in Herzberger, 2002; Groth, Marnat, 1990), and the way they understand violence or their identification with the role of a victim). The higher rate among young women with higher education who confirm the presence of violence in their environment may testify that the definition of violence is not fully understood by less educated women (Nowakowska, Jabłońska, 1998).

Gathering information about violence based on observers' reports also has its weak points. This method enables learning what others think about this topic, but because of the possible influence of common factors that bias beliefs about others (including, for instance, the illusory character of perceived correlations, liking or disliking, protecting and reinforcing "self"), data collected this way cannot be treated as fully trustworthy and true. For instance data obtained from children regarding domestic violence between their parents go way beyond the official statistics (Weis, 1989, as cited in Herzberger, 2002). Research results also indicate a very significant disproportion between women who themselves admit they were victims of violence and those who know other women that are victims. This may lead to an assumption that in Poland some women keep secret the fact that they are or were mistreated by their closest ones- particularly that the number of women who admit that they were victims of violence is lower in Polish studies than results from similar data from the West (Nowakowska, Jabłońska, 1998).

Retrospective data is also subject to errors, because people make mistakes when estimating frequency of events from the past. It is also difficult to precisely state when specific events took place (Herzberger, 2002). However, such difficulties do not disqualify attempts taken to evaluate domestic violence - they only indicate what caution has to be exercised during interpretation of the results.

In 2004, the Health Psychology Institute (IPZ) conducted a large research project aimed at determining the scale of domestic violence and offers of help addressed to its victims in Warsaw. General outcomes of the study indicate a relatively low social awareness-level regarding domestic violence. The majority of respondents accepted behaviors that are violent, because they perceived them differently (for instance slapping a 15-year-old son or daughter in the face, or insulting someone's partner). Some of the interviewees even thought that being violent at home from time to time is advisable and nobody should interfere. Only when the intensity of such behaviors becomes visible to the environment are they labeled as domestic violence and evaluated negatively (Kurza, 2005).

Almost half (47%) of Polish society is not able to imagine raising a child without hitting him and 78% of respondents agree that there are situations when the child has to be spanked (Roguska, 2008). Fifty-six percent of Poles think that parents too rarely physically punish their children (Nowakowska, Paluch, Zarębińska-Szczodry, 2001). Approximately 30% of children agree when asked whether there are situations when children should be spanked; 53% say spanking should be administered in case of robbery, 47% in case of alcohol usage, and 42% for smoking (Zakrzewska, 2001). A permissive attitude towards physical punishment of children is more often presented by men, older people (over 55), the lower educated and those living in villages (Roguska, 2008). At the same time, men, the oldest respondents (over 60), active Christian believers and those who claim they have central-right wing beliefs significantly rarely say violence towards children is common (Nowakowska, Paluch, Zarębińska-Szczodry, 2001). This probably is the same group of respondents who say that violence towards children does not include some forms of punishment. The majority of Poles who took part in the research project (60%) say that violence towards children has increased in recent years. However, the study conducted by Wenzel (2005, 2009) indicates that the number of parents who admit they hit their children has decreased. In 2005, 62% of parents with children under 19 said that their child had never been spanked; in 2009 this rate reached 69%. The inconsistency of the such results may be explained by the impact of media coverage of domestic violence topics. On the one hand this may lead to the easier noticing of such behaviors and thus to a conviction of its increased occurrence, while on the other hand, the condemning mood of media coverage may cause parents to treat their own behaviors as embarrassing. Decrease in support for an opinion that outsiders should intervene if they see a child being maltreated by parents (62 to 49%) is an interesting consequence of the social discussion about domestic violence. This decrease in support may result from fears related to threats of lawsuits against physical punishment and an overly rigorous perception or abuse of this right by people whose motives are not related to the child's welfare.

About one in eight Poles (12%) say that he/she has been hit at least once during quarrels by his/her partner. Eleven percent admit that they have hit their spouse. A small group of respondents (3%) experienced violence from adolescent children. One in nine adults admit experiencing violence from a different family member (for instance siblings, parents, grandparents). Over a third of the interviewed women (37%) declared in 2005 that they knew at least one woman beaten by her husband. In 2009 this rate decreased to 33% (Wenzel, 2005, 2009).

Twenty-seven percent in regular relations experiences insults, shouting and spoken aggression from their partners. From the interviewees' statements, it results that domestic violence is usually both-sided - those, who were victims of their partner's aggression, usually also used violence themselves. Women were victims a little more often than men and also more often admit they used violence (Wenzel, 2005, 2009).

The aforementioned project conducted by the Health Psychology Institute in Warsaw also included a study of professionals dealing with violence in their work. Teachers, healthcare employees, police, welfare workers and people giving psychological-pedagogic support participated. Their attitudes towards violence were studied, as well as their professional experience with victims of violence, their competence related to helping such people, and their subjective evaluation of working conditions. The replies given by healthcare employees, teachers and, to some extent, policemen revealed that some of them share the disadvantageous stereotypes that domestic violence may be justified in some cases (5.9%, 4.8% and 10.6% respectively) and that parents are free to choose their educational methods, including physical punishment (7.5%, 11.3% and 10.2%). These groups as well as employees of other services have less knowledge about violence and do not perceive its intensification (Riahi, 2005).

Research conducted within the “Childhood without violence” campaign revealed that part of the professionals working with families in which violence occurs think that “spanking” the child is justified in the following cases: if the child drinks alcohol (21%), robbery (17%), smoking cigarettes (13%), truancy (8%), lying and insubordination (7%), being late or damaging a valuable object (5%), poor grades (2%) (Zakrzewska, 2001). In research conducted the same year by IPZ, where healthcare employees, welfare workers, policemen, and municipal police as well as teachers from the Warsaw-Włochy region participated, as many as 40% of the respondents said that a child deserves spanking if it conducts petty robbery, 34% if it drinks alcohol and 25% if it shows disrespect towards its parents (Nikodemska, 2002). Policemensay that, among the professional categories, violence towards children is the least common (Nowakowska, Paluch, Zarębińska-Szczodry, 2001). Study held in 2004 in the Lubuskie region, the District Public Prosecutor's Office revealed that 77.2% of the prosecutors say that mothers and children are the most common victims of violence. Only one person from this professional group (out of 22 respondents in total) indicated that every family member may become a victim - including men (Chrzanowska, 2005).

Research also indicates a difference between members of individual professions regarding the frequency of intervening. Policemen interviewed by IPZ most often said that they intervene every time they meet a case of violence. One out of five medical professionals did not intervene in any cases of violence towards children and less than half of teachers admitted they always intervened when they met a case of a child harmed in its family. In all of those professional groups, there were people who never intervened when they met a case of violence (Riahi, 2005). In comparison, 88.5% of interviewed probation officers said they always intervene when they meet a case of a harmed child. A completely different situation may be found in cases of socio-therapists, where only 38% of respondents said they intervened in every such situation (Kurza, 2004). The necessity to isolate the child from parents who harm it in extreme situations was supported most often by welfare workers (92%) and least often by policemen (42%) (Nowakowska, Paluch, Zarębińska-Szczodry, 2001).

A study aimed at evaluating support provided to victims of violence by other professional groups was also conducted. For instance, probation officers evaluated the work of school educators as giving the best support (81% of probation officers thought that their support was effective), followed by welfare workers (65%), and they said that doctors are the worst in this area (23% of probation officers said that doctors did not help at all) (Kurza, 2004).

Healthcare professionals presented themselves as least competent in supporting violence victims. This was also the professional group in cases of which the smallest number of members would like to educate in this area more. Welfare workers were the group that wanted to participate in training about domestic violence the most - 84% of them expressed a will to participate, and 61% said they already participated in such training. Welfare workers were said to be the most competent professional group regarding support to violence victims. They were also motivated and willing to educate themselves. Simultaneously, as research results show, this group is the most exposed to professional burnout (Riahi, 2005). It may thus be assumed that employees with higher job seniority may be less willing to intervene in situations of violence when compared to those who have been on the job for only a few years.

Research conducted among welfare workers dealing with child protection in other countries (Howe, Herzberger, Tennen, 1988; Herzberger, 2003) indicated that they also evaluated punishment depending on their gender. Women-professionals said that parents' punishing behavior was more harsh than in men's opinions. Men-professionals evaluated physical punishment meted out by fathers as more harsh than meted out by mothers. The professionals also said that punishment of sons was more severe than punishment of daughters. Other research revealed that nurses more often said that a case was violent if the victim was a woman than if the victim was a man. Women dealing with psychical health said the same indicators (for instance children's sexual behavior) testified about abuse more so than men did (O'Toole, O'Toole, Webster & Lucal, 1994, as cited in Herzberger, 2003).

The presented results reveal significant differences in levels of social awareness regarding domestic violence between different social groups. This diversity may be a reason for a relatively frequent phenomenon of not noticing violence and, what follows, not helping victims - presented both by lay persons as well as by those, who, because of their profession or social role, are qualified to support violence victims.

Because only a few years have passed since welfare agencies in Poland received rights and duties related to counteracting domestic violence, the level of psychological knowledge about conditions of welfare workers' readiness to give support in situations of violence is still not high.

As results from a study held by Szczepańska (2008), 82% of Polish society expect the support of local authorities - communal and municipal welfare centers - in difficult situations. These expectations are not for just any help, but for effective support. And effective support depends largely on professional competence and skills for drafting new, appropriate strategies, resulting from constantly evolving scientific knowledge and experience (see Daro, Cohn, Donnelly, 2004). There is no data about the willingness to help presented by lay Poles.

This is why learning about conditions for readiness to intervene in domestic violence, both by social welfare workers as well as people not dealing professionally with support to others, and learning the meaning of factors that may condition this readiness, may increase social awareness in this area - increase willingness to actively counteract all forms of violence, and in consequence limit it.

Examples of concepts explaining support

Supporting behavior is usually understood as behavior aimed at giving some advantage to other people. The majority of theories explaining support were formulated in order to explain willingness to give help or forbear giving help in crisis situations - particularly in cases of sudden incidents that affect other, usually unknown, persons. It is impossible to present all the theoretical proposals offered by psychology in this article. We will thus briefly discuss only a few examples that present the general conditions for readiness to undertake support behavior.

Norm theories

Norm theories assume that helping others results from some social norms which people feel obliged to conform to. The norms, understood as socially agreed demands and prohibitions, internalized by individuals regarding desirable and undesirable behaviors in given situations, may be descriptive or obligational. Descriptive norms define how to behave, and acting according to them is said to be beneficial, effective and the most common in a given society. Obligational norms tell us what we should do in a given situation and are related to social approval or disapproval. Disapproval is usually linked to a number of sanctions executed by members of the social group to which the person who breaks the rules belongs. Behaving incompatibly with the norms in a situation in which somebody feels responsible for fulfilling them may also cause unpleasant intra-psychical consequences (for instance a feeling of guilt, or a disturbance in self-esteem).

The basic and oldest norms include prohibition of aggressiveness and requisition to help (related to responsibility and reciprocity norms), as well sex-related norms that not only regulate the sexual area, but also are the source of detailed rules for gender and type roles (Aronson. Wilson, Akert, 1997; Wojciszke, 2000; Dweyer, 2005).

The social responsibility norm demands helping people whose fate depends on us and who need help. The dependence of another person's fate on our actions increases the willingness to help - even if we do not profit from this, do not like the person, or if the person learns about our support only in the far future or never at all (Berkowitz, 1972).

The reciprocity norm, in general, commands helping persons who helped us in the past. This norm includes requisitioning help or doing a favor, that is, to accept support from others and requisitioning it by returning favor with favor (Gouldner, 1960, as cited in Zimbardo, Ruch, 1997). Reciprocation of support does not depend on liking the other person (Regan, 1971, as cited by Wojciszke, 2000).

Stimulation-balance model

Piliavin, Dovidio, Gaertner and Clark (1981), the creators of this model, assume that an observer seeing someone suffer aims at reducing the unpleasant emotions caused by viewing the that person's suffering. According to this model, supporting behavior depends on the strength of emotional stimulation caused by observing someone else's problems (and the strength increases as the situation becomes more unambiguous, longer-lasting and the closer the distance felt by the spectator towards the person who needs support), on how unpleasant the stimulation is, and whether reduction through supporting behavior means greater profit than cost.

Costs of support include for instance time, effort, and exposure to danger; and profits include increased feeling of one's own effectiveness and self-esteem, and other people's admiration. Costs related to forbearing support include self-blame, negative reaction from other people, and one's own suffering caused by the victim's suffering; and benefits include for instance the possibility to realize alternative goals. The stimulation-balance model assumes that when both costs of support and costs of forbearing support are small, behavior depends on what the spectator deems as normative for the situation. If the costs of support are high and costs of forbearance low, the observer usually would not intervene (denies the necessity to help, ignores it or abandons the situation). Giving support is the most probable if forbearance costs are high and support costs low. If both costs of support and forbearance are high, the spectator usually intervenes indirectly - for instance by calling a specialist or changing his subjective evaluation of the situation in order to decrease the costs of forbearance (denies the need for support, decreases the value of the victim, decreases one's own feeling of responsibility for the victim's fate, etc.) Research indicates that costs of giving support have a bigger impact on violence witnesses than costs of forbearance. Costs of forbearance affect behavior mainly if costs of support are low (Dovidio, 1984).

Researchers emphasize that if the victim suffers because of a natural catastrophe, witnesses usually sympathize with it. But when suffering is a result of man-made violence, the situation becomes more complex - in such cases costs of support may be particularly high (because there is a conflict of interests between victim and perpetrator) (Herman, 1998; Kubacka-Jasiecka, 2004; Obuchowski, 2000). Herman (1998, page 11) even emphasizes that "elimination from consciousness is a natural reaction to violence".

Empathy-altruism model

The empathy-altruism model , proposed by Bateson (1991), assumes that empathy felt by the spectator towards the person in trouble is the basic factor that induces people to take up supporting behavior. Empathic stimulation motivates one to help the victim regardless of whether it is in the spectator's interest, and even if his costs are higher than any possible benefits. Altruism induced by empathy is conducive to giving greater, more delicate and less whimsical support, leads to a decrease of aggressiveness and greater cooperation (Bateson, Ahmad, Stocks, 2008). According to Bateson, people may also help others when they do not feel empathy towards the person needing help, but in such cases the benefits connected to giving support usually have to be higher than the possible losses.

Motivation to help once empathy has been stimulated also has many limitations. Associating another person's expression (which should be appropriately sharp and intense) with one's own emotional state and experience is a condition that has to be met in order for the empathic reaction to occur (Reykowski, 1979; Hoffman, 2006). But even if empathic identification with the victim occurs, this will not necessarily lead to giving support. Pro-social motivation resulting from empathy may be subject to various limitations related to excessive empathic stimulation, cognitive mistakes (like the closeness mistake - mistaking one's own group, friendship, similarity) or the here-and-now mistake (Hoffman, 2006), as well as the life history of persons about to help. It does not address all needs, may lead to unmoral behaviors (for instance bias towards close ones), may cause harm both to the helping person and the person that is helped, and may lead to actions against the social good (Bateson, Ahmad, Stocks, 2008). The heightened feelings of empathy may be too weak to activate the ability to help - particularly in cases of persons raised in conditions of permanent stimulation by impulses causing pain. Feeling sympathy and compassion towards victims of violence who themselves conduct abuse may be a barrier in reacting effectively to violence. People who unintentionally identify with the sufferers may even be unable to conduct some professional roles that require effective protection of victims. Also people with unsolved or pathological identity problems (for instance consequences of traumatic experiences) may have difficulty in supporting others, in protecting or helping them (Kubacka-Jasiecka, 2004).

Decision crisis intervention model

This model was proposed by Latane and Darley (1970). Their study was inspired by an observation that the number of spectators of a critical event decreases the probability of giving support to the victim. According to the researchers, help is related to the necessary fulfillment of five conditions - and even if one of them is not fulfilled, actions toward the person needing support will be forborne.

Deciding about the possible intervention is done step by step:

I. Noticing the event.

A critical situation must first of all be noticed. The observer's hurriedness or contemplation may affect the noticing - haste makes us less interested in what is happening around us and thus decreases the probability to help another person. This factor is more important than personality factors (for instance the level of religiousness) (Darley, Batson, 1973).

II. Interpretation of the event as a crisis situation

Noticing the situation is not sufficient for intervention. The witness himself has to answer the question how serious the situation is and how necessary it is to help the person in need. Unambiguity of the situation is important - the more unclear the situation is, the more the witness is willing to search for indications in the behavior of other witnesses. Observers of a sudden event watch one another, and if they do not see any indications of anxiety or actions, they think that the situation does not require intervention (this phenomenon is called cumulation of ignorance or the ignorance of many) (Latany, Darley, 1970). Research revealed that the higher the number of witnesses are who watch a critical event, the lower the probability is that the victim will receive help. This dependency was named the phenomenon of the indifferent passer-by. This phenomenon disappears when the situation becomes unambiguous and cannot be interpreted other than as an accident (Latane, Darley, 1968).

III. Accepting responsibility

Interpretation of the observed situation as critical and requiring intervention is connected with the decision to accept personal responsibility for intervention and helping the victim. The number of witnesses and the conviction that someone has already intervened are the factors with key roles at this stage. If there are many witnesses of the accident, responsibility dispersion appears - because other people are present, the individual loses the feeling of personal responsibility for what is happening. Dispersion of responsibility decreases the personal costs of a specific behavior - for instance through a decrease in the feeling of guilt and shame (Kubacka-Jasiecka, 2004). However, some social roles may inhibit this phenomenon - for instance the role of group leader (Wojciszke, 2000). At this stage, the influence of people with authority or power may have a significant role. Subordination to regulations or orders releases us from our responsibility; thus acting under their influence may be stronger than the feeling of a just or individual value (Zimbardo, Ruch, 1997). Study results indicate that accidental witnesses have a stronger willingness to help in natural conditions than in laboratory conditions. This probably results from the passive role accepted by research subjects - renouncing responsibility in favor of the researcher and submitting to the experiment rules. Accepting responsibility would require a situation analysis that would activate norms and rules ordering helpful behavior, and turning control mechanisms on. A conflict of motives - between being convinced that there is a need to react and the will to avoid costs - may lead to transferring responsibility to others, manifested in the so-called endurance tactics, with the hope that someone will replace us (Kubacka-Jasiecka, 2004).

IV. Knowledge of the correct form of support and ability to provide it

Knowing what form of support is appropriate in a given situation and the ability to use it, are conducive to readiness to intervene in a crisis situation.

V. Deciding to help

Even if the observer of a critical event knows what form of support is correct, there may be some other circumstances that may prevent him from acting. He may be afraid of being ridiculed or of deteriorating the victim's situation by inappropriate actions. He may also be afraid for his own safety. Fear of being ridiculed weakens if the witnesses may discuss the observed event among themselves, settle on its meaning, discuss an action plan and explain the sense of the actions after they are finished.

The model prepared by Latane and Darley was created as a result of many studies that took into account both the fact that many intervention decisions are taken very fast - sometimes even automatically - as well as situations in which witnesses of a crisis situation have more time, enabling a detailed analysis of the whole situation and the role they may play in it. This aspect of the model corresponds to situations of support given both by welfare employees as well as people who do not deal professionally with helping others. The determination of decision stages done by Latane and Darley, as well as presentations of the possible impact on each of the stages, makes it possible to understand the basic conditions of readiness to intervene, and to introduce new variables to the model - for instance situational factors determining violence - that may turn out to have an important impact on the final decision made by observers of violence.

Purpose of the study

The purpose of the study was to compare the level of declared willingness to intervene in domestic violence by welfare workers and people not dealing professionally with helping others, as well as to check the impact of relations between victim and perpetrator and the type of violence on this willingness to intervene. Three basic study questions were formulated:

1. Are there differences in willingness to intervene in domestic violence cases between professionals who help in situations of violence and non-professionals who are not involved as a rule in such support?
2. What is the role of the initial decision stages (evaluation of violence level, feeling of responsibility and knowledge of the appropriate form of support) in evaluating the probability of intervention by welfare workers and people not dealing professionally with such support?
3. What is the impact of the type of violence and relation between participants on readiness to intervene in domestic violence cases?

The hypotheses were as follows:

1 Because of their profession (training and experience, but also because welfare workers were studied in their place of work), *readiness to intervene (in general and on each stage of decision-making) in cases of domestic violence should be higher among welfare workers than in the control group - people who do not deal professionally with helping others.*

2 *Knowledge should be the best predictor of intervention in the group of welfare workers, and in case of the control group - responsibility.* It may also be presumed that the role of evaluating violence levels may be different in both groups. If people who are not dealing professionally with support do evaluate their ability to help as worse and the situation of violence as more serious than they realized initially, they may desist from active help because of fear of failure or

wanting to avoid danger to themselves. However, welfare workers, because of their professional responsibilities, may try to intervene.

3 Three situational factors have an impact on readiness to intervene in situations of violence.

3.1Because of their competence and professional experience related to regular support given to violence victims and their families, *welfare workers will declare a similar level of readiness to intervene regardless of whether the perpetrator is a family member or an outside person (*hypothesis 3.1.a). *However, people who do not deal professionally with support,* because of the rule not to interfere in private lives of others, *will declare a greater readiness to help a person outside a family circle rather than another person within the same familiar (*hypothesis 3.1.b).

Type of violence should differentiate the readiness to help - *all subjects will be most ready to help victims of physical abuse (*because of its suggestiveness and unambiguity), *to a lesser degree victims of sexual abuse (*because of its controversy), *and least in cases of psychical violence.*

The method

Participants

The study was held in two groups: welfare workers and people not dealing professionally with helping others.

The target study group were welfare workers employed in the Municipal Welfare Center in Wrocław, who agreed to anonymously participate in the study. A total of 138 welfare workers decided to participate and 14 refused. In the study 120 questionnaires were used and 18 were rejected as inappropriately or incompletely filled in. The group of studied welfare workers consisted of 111 women and nine men, aged 23-54 (M=41.6), who have been working on this position for 1 to 32 years (M=14.7).

The control group consisted of adult Wrocław residents who do not deal professionally with helping others; they had secondary education or higher, and their ages were similar to the study group. A total of 148 people decided to participate; 21 refused, including four who refused during the tests. For analysis 120 questionnaires were used, and 28 were rejected as inappropriately or incompletely filled in. The group consisted of 61 women and 59 men, aged 20-60 (M=36.9).

Wrocław, one of the Poland's largest cities, seems interesting both because of the high number of social problems arising in big groups, and also because of the complex organization of the Municipal Welfare Center, thanks to which it has a number of bureaus characteristic of smaller units operating in other cities and villages. Furthermore, the Wrocław Municipal Welfare Center is one out of only a handful of such institutions that have introduced specialist units responsible for supporting welfare workers in solving specific social problems (including domestic violence, drug and alcohol addiction, and mental disorders).

Measures

Independent variables:

Two groups participated in the study: basic, including welfare workers; and control - people not dealing professionally with helping others. Variables related to the situation of violence included the type of violence (psychological, physical and sexual) and the type of relation between victim and perpetrator (family, when the perpetrator was a member of the victim's family - a person related by blood or marriage - or non-family, when an outside person was the perpetrator). In order to manipulate these factors, descriptions of violence situations were prepared, with a group of competent jurors validating their adequacy and clarity. In order to make the descriptions clear, unambiguous and relevant to actual situations as much as possible, each description, or story, contained not only a specific arrangement of the basic independent variables, i.e. the form of violence (3x) and relation between victim and perpetrator (2x), but also took into account the perpetrator's gender (woman, man), whose victim could be a woman, man or child (6x) and the victim's reaction (active, passive) (2x) (despite the fact that the two latter variables were not analyzed in this article). As a result, descriptions of 72 situations of violence were created. Examples of these stories are presented below.

> 1. In a compartment on a train enter a man and a girl about twelve. Without worrying about the rest of the passengers the man , loudly gesticulates to the accompanying child: "How terrible you look! Your dress is total rubbish! And how am I have to show you at this meeting? Nobody will treat me seriously with a daughter in a potato sack! Are you completely without taste?". The whole carriage can hear, as the little girl explains: "I'm sorry, I didn't want to upset you, I didn't know ... I'll make myself look better."
>
> 2. The sounds of a terrible scene are coming from Nowak's apartment. Finally the door opens and Mr. Nowak, in his pajamas, is followed out into

the stairwell by Mrs. Nowak, who is trying to push and kick her husband down the stairs. Mr. Nowak has a cut lip and flushed cheeks. He is screaming: “You’ll regret this! I’m going to call the police right away! People, help me!”

3. Edith and Dorothy are a pair of 26 year-old’s; they live together and raise Dorothy’s five year-old daughter. The previous evening they went to the cinema, and then ate dinner at a restaurant. After returning home, Edith was tired and wanted to go to sleep, but Dorothy had hopes of making love with her. Despite Edith’s express refusal, Dorothy by force and threats of leaving forced her to have intercourse. Next day Edith, telling about this incident to her sister, said, “I almost did not defend myself, because I care about her too much to do anything, And... frankly speaking, nothing had happened”.

Dependant variables:

According to the model prepared by Latane and Darley, readiness to intervene is understood as a process characterized by five consecutive stages leading to a declaration of help or omission. The stages are as follows:

- noticing the event
- evaluating the level of violence
- evaluating the level of one’s own responsibility to react
- evaluating one’s own knowledge regarding the possibility to help
- evaluating the probability of one’s own reaction

The accepted dependant variables referred to the stages of intervention decisions - with omission of the first stage (noticing the event).

The subjects’ task was to relate to each story by using four questions: evaluation of level of violence (conviction that it requires intervention), level of one’s own responsibility to react, level of knowledge about the appropriate form of help, and evaluation of the probability to intervene in the situation. The subjects used a scale of 1 to 5, with 1 meaning the lowest level of appropriate variables and 5 - the highest level.

In this article, the impact of situational variables on the general readiness to help and on individual stages of the process is analyzed.

Procedure

The study was held on the premises of the Wrocław Municipal Welfare Center, at the headquarters of the Field Welfare Teams. Each participant filled in the tests during work hours, at his or her desk, in silence, in the presence of members of the same team and the researcher. Control group members received questionnaires by e-mail and sent them back the same way after filling them in, or filled them in during direct contact with a researcher.

The subjects' task was to relate to six different situations of violence (described in a story) by answering four questions formulated for each of the situations. The questions referred to the stages of taking intervention decisions in crisis situations. Using a five-point scale, the subjects selected a digit that reflected their opinion in the given situation to the highest degree.

All 72 stories were divided into six groups in order to make it possible for each participant to refer to each type of violence (3x), with the perpetrator being both a family member and an outsider (2x). Each group contained 12 different descriptive situations, differing by characteristics of the participating people (who is using violence against whom - 6x - and the victim's reaction of- 2x). Selection of situation sets for each participant consisted in randomly selecting one out of 12 possible descriptions from each of the six initial groups.

Results

The data obtained was analyzed using variation analysis with repeated measures: 2 relations between victim and perpetrator (family, outsider) x 3 forms of violence (psychological, physical, sexual) x 4 stages of decision making (evaluation of the violence level, one's own responsibility, knowledge of the appropriate form of help, probability to intervene); inter-group analysis x 2 groups (welfare workers, people not dealing professionally with helping others); and inter-group analysis (Table 1). The NIR Fisher test was used in the post-hoc analysis. Variation analysis made it possible to evaluate the level of readiness of welfare workers and non-professional persons, and to compare both groups in this area (the first study question). It also revealed the impact of the form of violence and the relation between victim and perpetrator on the readiness level (third question). In order to find the answer to the second question, regression analysis was used; this made it possible to evaluate the share of individual decision taking stages in the final declared probability level for intervening in violence situations.

Variance analysis proved the significance of all the independent variables taken into account in the study. Simple effects, related to the general readiness of the participants to intervene, were obtained for all variables except for the relation between victim and perpetrator (family member or an outsider as the perpetrator). This last variable turned out to be significant for its interaction effects. The conducted analysis also revealed different meanings of violence variables in the individual stages of deciding about domestic violence.

Table 11-1. Variance analysis with repeated measurement [replace commas with points throughout the Table]

	SS	df	MS	F	p
	69722.50	1	69722.5	7219.229	0.001
{1}GROUP	228.01	1	228.01	23.608	0,001
Error	2298.58	238	9.66		
{2}RELATION	0.12	1	0.12	0.051	0,822
RELATION*GROUP	12.84	1	12,84	5.570	0,019
Error	548.79	238	2.31		
{3}VIOLENCE	1438.88	2	719.44	226.685	0,001
VIOLENCE*GROUP	9.84	2	4.92	1.551	0,213
Error	1510.70	476	3,17		
{4}READINESS	909.47	3	303.16	296.638	0,001
READINESS*GROUP	3.42	3	1.14	1.117	0,341
Error	729.69	714	1.02		
RELATION*VIOLENCE	9.45	2	4.73	1.488	0,227
RELATION*VIOLENCE* GROUP	6.41	2	3.21	1.010	0,365
Error	1511.88	476	3.18		
RELATION*READINESS	2.22	3	0.74	2.393	0,067
RELATION*READINESS* GROUP	1.05	3	0.35	1.136	0,334
Error	220.65	714	0.31		
VIOLENCE*READINESS	86.85	6	14.47	30.811	0,001
VIOLENCE*READINESS* GROUP	5.22	6	0.87	1.854	0,086
Error	670.85	1428	0.47		
RELATION* VIOLENCE* READINESS	10.09	6	1.68	4.629	0,001
2*3*4*1	3.53	6	0.59	1.619	0,138
Error	518.96	1428	0.36		

Readiness to intervene in situations of domestic violence by welfare workers and people not dealing professionally with helping others

As predicted (hypothesis 1), welfare workers declare a higher general readiness to intervene (M=3.68) compared to people not dealing professionally with helping others (M=3.28; F(1.236)=23.36; p=.001).

The correctness of this hypothesis is also confirmed by analysis results regarding individual steps of intervention decision making (Table 11-2).

Table 11-2. Comparison of readiness level to intervene in situations of domestic violence between welfare workers and people not dealing professionally with helping in situations of violence

Stages of readiness to intervene	Welfare workers		Control group		
	M	SD	M	SD	
Level of violence	4.33	.15	3.99	.15	-3.94***
Responsibility	3.57	.16	3.10	.16	-4.91***
Knowledge	3.47	.17	3.07	.17	-4.05***
Probability of intervention	3.35	.16	2.97	.16	-3.95***

Note *$p<.05$; **$p<.01$; ***$p<.001$

They also indicate a similar pattern of relating to situations of violence at each stage of decision making presented by both study groups. All participants evaluate the level of violence they witnessed at the highest. Their own feeling of responsibility to intervene and knowledge of the appropriate of form of support were evaluated significantly lower (p< .001 in both groups). Probability of intervention was evaluated the lowest (the difference between second and third and the fourth decision stage in both groups at p< .05 level of significance). Results of this analysis prove that if a situation of violence is noticed (and in the study this condition was met because all the participants related to descriptions of specific situations), it is usually judged as requiring intervention. On the other hand, high marks in evaluating the level of violence, indicating the necessity to intervene, are greatly disproportionate to one's own responsibility for taking such actions, as well as knowledge of adequate forms of support and the probability of possible witnesses participating in active opposition to the violence. These results testify to the complexity of the process leading to intervention in situations of violence. They suggest a different meaning of the individual decision making stages in evaluating the probability to intervene, and maybe also the influence of other factors not included in the Latane and Darley model - for instance variables describing the situation of violence itself.

The relation between the victim and perpetrator is another factor. Although this relation does not differentiate the general readiness to intervene, welfare workers are more willing to help the victim if the perpetrator is a member of his family (M=3.72) rather than an outsider (M=3.63). People who do not deal professionally with helping others declare a higher general readiness to act when the perpetrator is an outsider (M=3.34) than when it is a family member (M=3.23; F (1.238)=5.570; p= .019). These results have confirmed hypothesis 3.1.b, but did not confirm hypothesis 3.1.a.

In order to check what the share is of individual stages of decision-making in the final decision to intervene, adequate multiple regression analyses were conducted for each of the tested groups (i.e. welfare workers and people not dealing professionally with helping others). Table 3 presents the results of the analyses. As predicted, knowledge of appropriate forms of support (knowledge) turned out to be the best predictor of the probability to intervene in the case of welfare workers. In the case of persons not dealing professionally with helping others - feeling of responsibility to intervene was the best predictor. The fact that welfare workers took into account not only the moral choice, but first of all their competence, might be a result of the study conditions - the topic was directly related to their professional activity and they were replying in their place of work and during work hours. These factors could have activated their image of themselves as employees of Municipal Welfare Centers, expected by their clients and superiors to take up effective actions in situations requiring them to do so. Effectiveness is strongly related to competence; knowledge of appropriate forms of help turned out to be the strongest predictor of the declared probability to intervene. The role played by the level of observed violence also seems interesting. The results clearly prove that normal witnesses of violence, when considering their active opposition to violence taking place, to a higher degree take into account the costs they may incur. Welfare workers, who, because of their profession, probably feel obliged to intervene (and definitely to declare intervention) in situations that are also dangerous to them.

Table 11-3. Summary of the independent variable regression: "Probability of intervention" in the study groups.

Variables	Beata	T (116)	p
Welfare workers R square =.820 (F(3,116)=176,59; p<.001			
Level of violence	-.085	-1.839	.068
Responsibility	..382	5.383	.001
Knowledge	.608	8.501	.001
Control group - R square =.812 (F(3,116)=166,72; p<.001			
Level of violence	-.113	-2.113	.037
Responsibility	.610	9..902	.001
Knowledge	.439	7.464	.001

Readiness to intervene and the type of violence used by the perpetrator

The type of violence significantly influences the participants' general readiness to help the victim. The highest level of readiness was declared in cases of physical violence (M=4.11), weaker in sexual violence (M=3,44) and weakest in psychological violence (M=2.89; F(2.472)=231.15; p= .001) (hypothesis 3.2). This hypothesis was also proved in cases of readiness to help on each of the decision making process stages.

The type of observed violence has an impact on the stages of intervention - in cases of all types of violence, the evaluations of violence levels of are highest when compared to evaluations done on the next stages of the decision process (for all types of violence p<.001). However, in cases of physical and sexual violence, the feeling of responsibility to help is higher than knowledge about appropriate forms of support (for both types of violence p<.001), and the probability of helping is adequate to the evaluation of competence (in cases of physical violence p<.962 and sexual violence p<.172). In cases of psychological violence, the witnesses feel less responsible to intervene despite the conviction that they have knowledge that would solve the problem (p<.001). In such cases they also declare the lowest probability of actions (for all types of violence and all stages of the decision process p<.001). Readiness to intervene in such cases is similar to the responsibility they feel toward this situation.

The course of the intervention depends also on who the perpetrator is. In cases of psychological violence, the feeling of responsibility is significantly weaker if the perpetrator is a member of the victim's family than if it is an outside person (M=2.60 and M=2.75 respectively, p< .001).

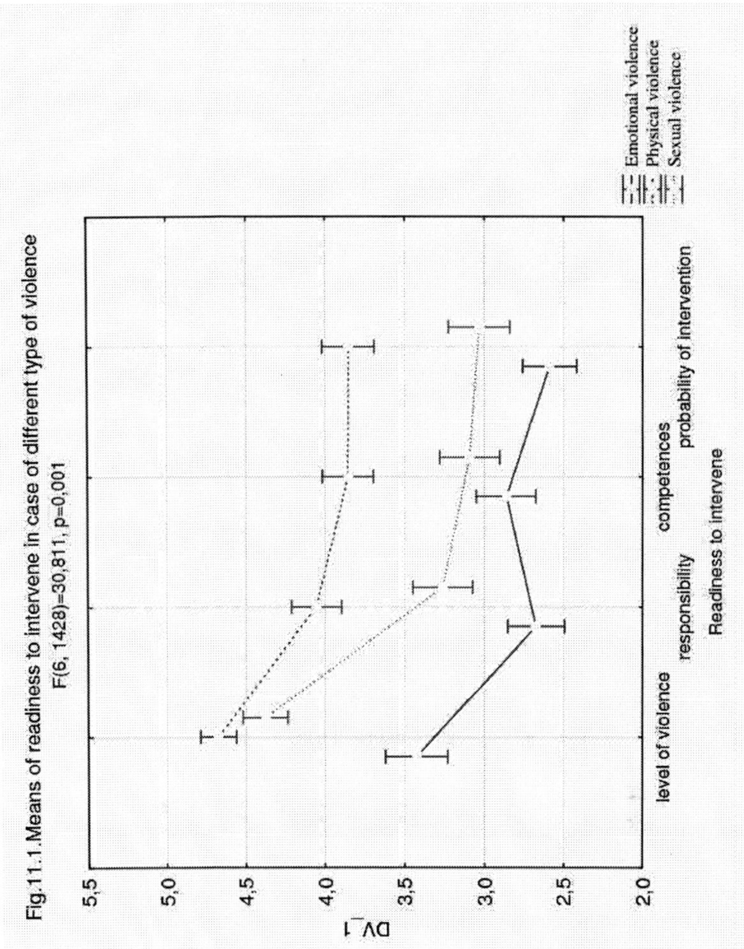

Fig.11.1.Means of readiness to intervene in case of different type of violence

Fig.11.2. Means of readiness to intervene in case of different type of violence and relation between victim and perpetrator

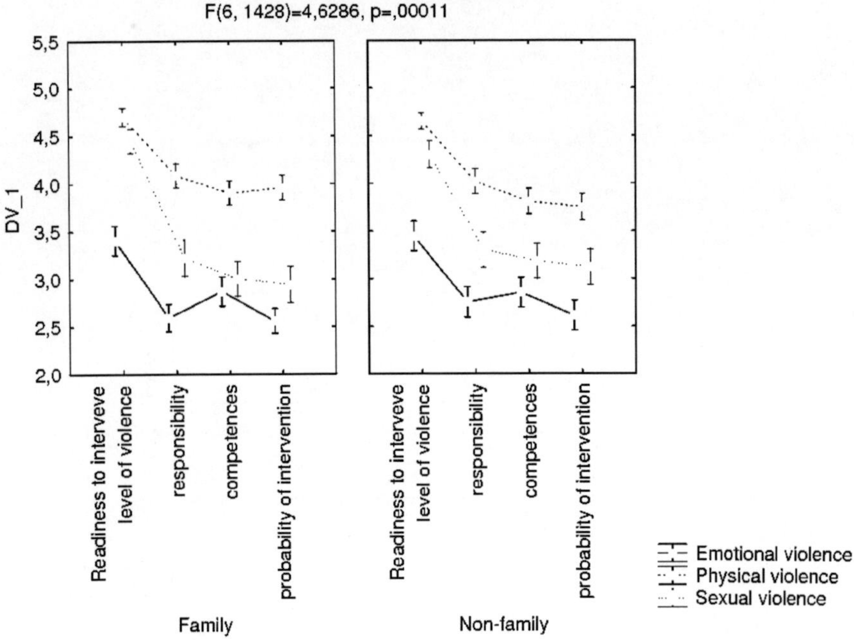

In cases of physical violence, the relation between the victim and the perpetrator has no impact on the feeling of responsibility or evaluation of one's own competence, but affects the final decision related to the probability of intervention. All participants were inclined toward greater activity if the perpetrator was a member of the family than if it was an outside person (M=3.96 and M=3.75 respectively, p< .01).

However, the highest meaning of the relation between victim and perpetrator was observed in cases of sexual violence. All participants said that such violence, caused by a family member, is more serious and requires intervention compared to a situation in which it is caused by an outside person (M=4.45 and M=4.30 respectively, p< .001). However, they evaluated their competence (M=3.18 and M=3.00; p< .001) and probability to help (M=3.12 and M=2.94; p< .001) greater when they considered an outside person as the perpetrator than when a family member was the assailant.

Discussion of the results

Readiness to intervene in cases of domestic violence presented by welfare workers and people not dealing professionally with helping others

The conducted research demonstrated that welfare workers declare a higher readiness to intervene in crisis situations than people not dealing professionally with helping others (hypothesis 1). Knowledge of appropriate forms of action is the strongest predictor of probability to help the victim by welfare workers; and among people not dealing professionally with helping others, it is feeling a sense of responsibility (hypothesis 2).

Welfare workers are one of the so-called "first contact" professional groups (other such groups include probation officers, health care workers and the police) - professionals working directly with the client or patient and his or her family. One of the welfare workers' basic tasks (specified in legal actions regulating welfare and counteracting domestic violence) is helping families where violence occurs. So, for this professional group, reacting to violence is not only a question of morality or personal choice (and this is how the decision to help or desist from helping may be described in the case of the control group), but also a legally binding duty. The particular importance (and thus the expectations of other professional groups) of this professional group in preventing and counteracting domestic violence is emphasized by the fact that welfare workers, because of their relatively regular and direct contact with the family, may act as coordinators of team efforts, as a link between institutions caring for the family. This particular role of the welfare worker would explain his higher readiness to declare help in cases of violence compared to the control group.

Simultaneously, welfare workers (particularly employees of the Wrocław Municipal Welfare Center - the study group) are a relatively well trained group (there were many internal training sessions during 2004-2006 and then as part of the "Versatile education - effective support" project in 2007). This group not only more eagerly participates in training sessions (seminars, conferences) regarding domestic violence than the other "first contact" professional groups, but also perceives the highest meaning of such sessions (OBOP, 2007). Because such training also includes definitions and types of violence, welfare workers might recognize violence more easily and more often than the control group members. After learning about how to help during such training, welfare workers might also feel more competent to help, as well as more responsible - as professionals trained to help. Taking into account that knowledge of appropriate forms of help is in their case the main predictor of probability to intervene, study results confirm the importance of training , as one of the most effective methods in counteracting violence. It is also worth remembering that obligations resulting from the professional role they fulfill, as well as sound preparation for reacting to violence , may make the costs of desisting from help higher in the case of welfare workers than in the case of the control group (for instance the expectations of the environment or their superiors or greater feelings of guilt resulting from obligations to their profession).

However, we cannot forget about the impact of social expectations towards the profession of welfare workers on auto-presentation of the participants. The study included only declarations of help, not actual behavior. Welfare workers might declare a higher readiness to help than members of the control group in order to fulfill their own expectations and not expose themselves to criticism of their professional competence.

The study of differences in declared readiness to intervene supplement assumptions of the theoretical model and facilitate practical use of the violence-prevention model. It turns out that being a welfare worker predisposes a witness to greater openness to help others. Assuming that the welfare workers' more frequent declaration of readiness to intervene results from their professional training to react in such violence situations, we may conclude that it is possible to increase the motivation that people have to help. The order of processes leading to intervention, described by Latane and Darley, would indicate the scope of important topics, covering which would significantly improve the effectiveness of educational projects (for instance education regarding violence recognition that requires reaction and/or teaching people effective methods of support).

Impact of relation type between victim and perpetrator on readiness to help

The relation between victim and perpetrator did not have impact on the overall readiness of study participants to intervene in crisis situations. However, it turned out to be an important determinant for the level of readiness of both groups. Contrary to predictions (hypothesis 3.1.a), welfare workers declared a higher readiness to help a victim who they thought was attacked by someone related by blood or marriage than one attacked by an outside person. Whereas, people not dealing professionally with helping others, in accordance with the assumptions, declared a higher readiness to intervene when the perpetrator was an outsider than if it was a family member (hypothesis 3.1.b).

The welfare workers' declaration of higher readiness to help victims assaulted by their family members rather than those attacked by outside persons could be explained by the update of one's image as a professional welfare worker. The fact that the study was held in the subjects' workplace (the Wrocław Municipal Welfare Center), during their work hours and in the presence of their co-workers, could support the correctness of this explanation. According to the hypothesis of social context primacy (Markus and Kunda, 1986, as cited by: Forgas, Wiliams, Wheeler, 2005), the concept of "self" currently available in operational memory is impacted by the social situation in which the person currently is. The part of the self image which is more cognitively available at the given moment determines the self-explanation process and is superior to other images of self. Thus it is probable that characteristics of the situation in which the welfare workers were, determined their way of thinking about themselves as persons whose job it is to help people. And to help the people they are supposed to help because of their profession.

In recent years, significant changes have been introduced into the welfare system, regarding helping families where violence occurs. In such cases, thanks to the Act of Counteracting Domestic Violence having been accepted, the family has the right to receive help. The Act imposes the duty on welfare workers, among others, to help people affected by domestic violence and describes methods of support. Moreover, another recently approved modification has put social work (as support in reinforcing or regaining the ability to function in society) as second among the most important tasks of welfare support. This emphasized the welfare workers' duty to help families not only financially. In order to address the new expectations, the Wrocław Municipal Welfare Center organized a series of internal training sessions regarding domestic violence. All these changes may have influenced a new way of perceiving domestic violence by welfare workers, through increasing their sensitivity to domestic violence, increasing their feeling of responsibility to help, and increasing their competence to help. This fact may also explain why welfare workers more highly evaluated their feelings of responsibility to react, as well as their competence to help and probability to react, when violence took place within a family.

The higher readiness to intervene in situations where the perpetrator was an outside person, as declared by people not dealing professionally with helping others, may be explained by the social norm not to interfere in another person's private life. This norm enables one to avoid empathy with victims of domestic violence (Bateson, Ahmad, Stocks, 2008) and protects against a feeling of responsibility, which, as the presented study indicated, is the main predictor of probability to intervene. The correctness of such an explanation is confirmed by the previously-mentioned decrease in Polish social opinion for legally prohibiting corporal punishment on children.

Impact of type of violence on readiness to intervene

The presented study demonstrated that all participants declare the highest readiness to help a victim of physical violence, lower if the violence is sexual, and lowest if it is psychological (hypothesis 3.2).

With the highest marks, as compared to sexual or psychological violence, being reserved for , the feeling of responsibility as well as knowledge of the appropriate way to help and the probability to intervene have two most important reasons. Firstly, physical violence is connected with the oldest and thus probably the most strongly internalized social norms regarding prohibition to do harm; it is usually identified with various physical actions resulting in injury and threat or in loss of life (also dictionary definitions of violence prove this), as well as with the responsibility norm. Secondly, because of its behavioral aspect and results, physical violence seems the most expressive, unambiguous and least controversial. The correctness of these explanations is confirmed by the fact that mainly cases of physical violence are reported to the authorities - psychological violence is reported very rarely. Such reporting occurs because physical violence usually results in bodily injury, which may be proven by forensic examination, a doctor's certificate or even a photo of the injury. It is also easier to be noticed and observed. In the case of physical violence we usually have specific actions and their results, which can simply be described. However, it should be remembered that for many types of social services, these specific facts are the basis for starting support actions. It is much more difficult to describe cases of psychological (Obuchowska, 1989) or sexual (Muehlenhard, Petersom, 2008) violence.

Emotional abuse is very difficult to quantify and it is also difficult to determine its intensity. The lack of literature regarding psychological violence proves the difficulty with such evaluation (Browne and Hervert, 1999). The same verbal communication, reaction, or activity in one situation may be completely neutral in another - yet be a big blow to the victim's psyche. Even the categories of psychological ill-treatment listed by Amnesty International (for instance imposing one's own judgments, or using verbal degradation) are so unclear, that they may include almost all types of unfair behavior. Difficulty in unambiguous evaluations of psychological violence and the norm of not interfering in the private lives of others may lead to a lesser feeling of responsibility to react in such situations. This was also reflected in the results of our study - they indicate that in situations of psychological violence, witnesses feel less responsible to react despite the conviction that they have the knowledge to solve the problem. They also declare the smallest probability for undertaking active measures in order to solve the problem. These dependencies apply mainly to situations in which the perpetrator is a member of the victim's family.

Emotional violence is a form of abuse that may appear in veiled form - for instance under the cover of reliability or caring for social norms: The perpetrator may, for instance, accuse the victim of behaving against social expectations (poor hygiene or wearing inappropriate clothes). Such a transfer of responsibility to the victim may result in the victim, as well as external witnesses, not perceiving the situation as violent. Some authors even notice that psychological violence is often difficult to differentiate from a regular quarrel (Badura-Madej, Dobrzyńska-Masterhazy, 2000). Other researchers dealing with the problem of violence in school, emphasize that some forms of psychological violence (for instance not allowing a student to join in discussions, imposing the "only correct" opinions on others, etc.) are socially accepted. This may result from the rather common conviction that teaching means giving unalterable, absolute truths to those who do not have requisite knowledge. Such forms of violence may be used for example by a teacher, completely unwillingly (Obuchowska, 1989).

Some professionals dealing with the problem of psychological violence pay attention to the fact that in some environments, as in school, the word "violence" is avoided (the word has negative emotional associations) and replaced by such euphemisms as "teasing" or, more recently, "mobbing". Such an operation decreases the meaning of the problem and may "normalize" it, leading to disrespect (Babicka, www.szkolabezprzemocy.pl).

Psychotherapists and other persons running violence workshops indicate that many clients are unaware what psychological violence is (Osipczuk, www.e-lama.pl, Drzewiecka, http://theppd.org/index.php?id=37,111,0,0,1,0).

When compared with physical violence, sexual abuse also seems to be belittled. Although the topic is relatively often mentioned in the media, disclosed facts about sexually-related assaults are often mockingly commented on - particularly if politicians are participating (for instance the famous scandal of December 2005, when the question "How can you rape a prostitute?" was posed in public). Arguments belittling sexual violence may serve various purposes - as in creating so-called "moral panic" - if they are used as an emotional-moral basis for debates on aggravation of punishment for perpetrators. As a result, public opinion notices only the particularly brutal or repulsive cases of sexual abuse, with the less "spectacular", but more often, cases not attracting such attention (Zadumińska, 2006).

The ambiguous and controversial character of sexual violence is also indicated by many studies dealing with the difficulty that external observers, victims, perpetrators and the law have in evaluating sexual behaviors as violent, as well as the attempts at theoretical conceptualization of this phenomenon undertaken by researchers (Muehlenhard, Petersom, 2008). Moreover, as results from the present study indicate, recognition of sexual violence itself, as well as evaluating a situation to determine if intervention is required, does not translate in a simple way into probability of intervention. All participants in this study acknowledged that this type of violence, if caused by a family member rather than an outside person, is more serious and requires intervention. However, they evaluated their competence and probability of helping the victims as higher when sexual violence was caused by an outside person.

Limitations

The conducted study has a few weak points:

- the study concerned only the declared readiness of participants to intervene in situations of violence, not their actual behaviors in such situations,
- readiness was measured by outright questions, giving the possibility for biased replies,
- the welfare workers were asked in their workplace, during their work, which might have had impact on their replies to the questionnaire,
- the described situations of violence differed according to the specific character's behavior , the place where the incident occurred, and the observer's distance, all of which might have had an impact on the accuracy of results for types of violence.

Summary

Despite the aforementioned weaknesses, the study enabled us to answer all the study questions. Among other things, the study proved that the witness's profession as welfare worker may predispose him to greater openness to help in domestic violence situations. Assuming that the welfare workers' declaration of will to intervene in cases of violence results from professional training, it may be concluded that it is possible to reinforce their readiness to help. The study, conducted within the Latane and Darley model, indicates the range of important topics which, if taken up, may significantly increase the effectiveness of educational projects. Such projects should concentrate not only on identifying violence as an event that requires social reaction, but should, first of all, give knowledge about effective methods for helping and skills that would enable the best possible use of this knowledge. On the other hand, the higher readiness to help if the perpetrator is a family member rather than an outsider seems alarming. It suggests that the social workers' readiness to counteract violence results only from their professional duties and is limited to those clients to which their professional activities apply. In order to understand how social workers thinks, as well as how to make educational activities more effective , it seems very important to study this issue in conditions different from those created in the present study. The relation between victim and perpetrator, as well as type of violence, on the process of deciding whether to intervene in a crisis, also indicates the necessity to include support activities into educational projects. Learning about factors that are conducive to helping or inhibiting one's readiness to assist would give a better understanding of violence and one's own behavior in such situations.

CHAPTER TWELVE

MULTIFACETED INTEGRATIVE THERAPY FOLLOWING CHRONIC CHILDHOOD TRAUMA

AGNIESZKA WIDERA-WYSOCZAŃSKA

Trauma has been with mankind from its beginning and has taken on the form of natural disasters, or those caused by man including various kinds of domestic violence. The therapy discussed here concerns a person's response to interpersonal chronic and complex trauma experienced in the family and in her or his immediate environment. Response to such trauma is very complex; thus in recent years a spate of systems has emerged to diagnose such persons, and various specific approaches have been developed. Some of the many which have influenced the method described here are the retrospective incest therapy of Christine Courtois (1998, Courtois, Ford, 2009), the therapy described by Pearlman (Pearlman, 2003; Pearlman, Courtois, 2005), the trauma therapy of John Briere (1992, Briere; Scott, 2006), solution-focused therapy and Ericksonian hypnosis for adult survivors (Dolan, 1991), as well as a sensorimotor and body approach to psychotherapy (Ogden, Minton, Pain, 2006; also Levine, 2005; Rothschild, 2000).

The retrospective therapy of Ch. Courtois was created in order to help women who experienced incestuous violence during childhood. Pearlman's therapy and Briere's trauma therapy are approaches applied to adults who experienced various types of childhood violence. The principal purpose of these approaches is to continue the person's development by triggering and applying the person's inner resources of a given traumatic experience and allowing that person to go beyond the actual level of operation. These are linguistic models of therapy based on a belief that narration is a phenomenon that can open up change that focuses around meanings applied to a given reality. They were defined by Ogden (Ogden, Minton, Pain, 2006) as a "top-down" approach according to which changes in the perceptions and emotions that occurred during the process of narrative expression lead to changes in bodily experiences, which in consequence leads to healing.

Solution-focused therapy and the Ericksonian hypnosis described by Dolan, targeted persons following childhood abuse, particularly sexual. Their overall purpose is to bring about stabilization and relief with reference to the symptoms experienced, as well as triggering and actively using the client's current resources in order to build a sound and satisfactory orientation towards the future. The result is a pattern of behavior without the earlier symptoms. Body-focused therapy described by Rothschild or Ogden, Minton, and Pain as well as by Levine is effective in working with people after traumas suffered in childhood. It is also effective in solving other problems that have resulted from childhood, including non-traumatic family-dynamics, which influence the personalities of the family members and the relationships with people. The purpose of this approach is for the person to cope with the traumatic past and help the client in building and experiencing an integrated feeling of self, based not only on imagination, thoughts and emotions but also on bodily feelings. This is a group of approaches described as "bottom-up" (after: Ogden, Minton, Pain, 2006), which recognizes that accessing the person's inner resources and working with their body contributes to a change in cognitive and emotional processes. I have noticed that one group of these methods pays particular attention to bringing out resources from the client's subconsciousness and using them to cope with the traumatic consequences and to build a good future. That group also includes solution-focused therapy, the approach of Milton Erickson as well as Neuro-Linguistic Programming. The other group of these methods focuses on reducing symptoms in the body in order to bring about positive changes in the person's emotional and cognitive processes.

In this paper the integrative "life-span" approach will be presented. This is an approach that has been emerging since 1987 in the Center for Therapy of People from Dysfunctional Families. Its basis consists of experiences of the present author and her collaborators in doing therapy with people who underwent traumas during childhood (grown-up children of alcoholics, grown-up children from dysfunctional families, persons after sexual abuse, and perpetrators of domestic violence).

Below I will describe the multifacetedness of this approach, focusing on who and what is covered by this integrative "life-span" therapy; what phenomena undergo diagnosis; what the assumptions are concerning the philosophy and methods of this approach; what its objectives and healing stages are with respect to the process and to the form; and what the traps are that may occur in the healing process. I will also present methods that emerge to monitor the efficiency of that healing.

Subject and object of integrative "live-span" psychotherapy for people after chronic trauma

The approach described is designed for adult persons who have undergone interpersonal, complex, chronic trauma during childhood, youth or adult life, as well as for their partners and children.

The object of the therapy is to deal with complex and chronic traumatic experiences (the description of features is to be found in Chapters 1 and 2) which cover different kinds of violence and neglect that take place in the family and environment.

The subject of the therapy is grown-up people and children who bear consequences as a result of undergoing interpersonal traumas. Thus the therapeutic procedure presented here covers at least two generations: parents and partners as well as their children. The inclusion of partners into the therapeutic process serves to build secure and functional relations with the close, familial ones and in this way creates an environment conducive to a patient's healing. A grown-up person reviews how experiencing relations between them (her or him) and their parents and those between the parents themselves) has influenced them in creating a model of connections which affects the quality of current relations. Therapeutic care also covers the client's children who have experienced domestic violence as a result of its intergenerational transmission. Adults owing to the increase of awareness of the past and through the work on their parental skills, build more secure connections between themselves and their child. Then the child can return to health more effectively and develop under better conditions.

During their own therapy, adults deal thus with their own life from the perspective of being their parents' child, from the perspective of being another adult's partner of, and from the perspective of being a parent (a caretaker) of their own children (Tab. 12-1).

Table 12-1. Subjects of integrative therapy for people after chronic trauma - various perspectives

Subjects of therapy - three generations	Objective - various perspectives
grown-ups who experienced complex chronic trauma during childhood, youth or adult life	deal with their own life from three perspectives: - being a child of their parents - being a partner of an adult - being a parent/caretaker for their children the grown-up deals with her/his life from two perspectives: -survivor's: adult as a person having been hurt in childhood and being hurt in adult life by their partner (and other people) -offender's: a person who in adult life hurts other people, her/his children and partners in particular
partners of grown-up clients	inclusion of partners helps to build: - safe and functional mutual relationships - creates an environment conducive to the healing of the patient and their children
children of grown-up clients	- work with children in connection with consequences they bear because of having experienced domestic violence as a result of its intergenerational transmission - work on parental skills to build secure connections between them and their child
parents of grown-up clients (the family of origin)	- Build current, functional, adult relationships if at all possible

The main goals of "life-span" psychotherapy

The overall purposes of life-span psychotherapy are to help the person rather than the family. No stress is put on modifying family relationships to keep the family together at any cost. On the contrary, the person is helped to regain their inner strength, their quality of life is increased, their security reinforced, and their inner and other resources rebuilt as are the sense of value, independence, the feeling of sound responsibility and adequate control.

It is important to rebuild contact with inner feelings, thoughts and skills that enable the client to regain confidence in their intuitions, which become tools to achieve goals and make changes in their current and future life. This is to be brought about by achieving such sub-objectives as becoming more aware of violence experienced and of the consequences resulting from and in connection with growing up in a dysfunctional family; breaking the bonds of silence and isolation; recognizing toxic roles, principles, and relationships within oneself and the environment, and learning new roles, values, and healthier relationships with relatives and others; creating a lifestyle free from dependence on parents, with whom relations to this point have had a "childish character", and from this point on to build a "grown-up relation"; and building a life free from the toxic partner, if abuse exists in the current family life, as is usually the case.

The premises underlying the "life-span" integrative therapy

The philosophy of the life-span approach is based on feminist theories (Brickman, 1984; Brownmiller, 1975; Rush, 1977); the theory of post-traumatic stress disorder (Briere, 1992; Briere, Scott, 2006; Figley, 1985; Herman, 1982); the theory of attachment (Bowlby, 1979, 1980, 1988) and the psycho-social development of Erik Erikson (1980). Additionally it reaches out to postulates of humanistic approaches, Milton Erickson (Dolan, 1991) and the neurolinguistic method (McDermott, Jago, 2006).

A psychotherapy that concerns traumas from childhood requires correct recognition of the dynamics of human development from birth to death. Thus the interactions of life-span psychotherapy include three time perspectives: we deal with the past of people hurt in order for them to be able to create their present and to build a functional future. The psychotherapist and the patient refer to the past trauma in order to find out about the causes of current problems and their impact on current and future life. An analysis of the past alone, however, is not enough to build a healthy life in the present. We deal with the present so that the person solves current problems that result from the past and learns a new mode of functioning in different spheres of life. We consider the future so that the person can plan their life, set goals, and foresee ways of their realization. Such therapy that reaches into the lives of an individual and their family from the past to the present in the approach presented is called "*life-span*".

Violence exists - it is a truth, not a fantasy by a child or a woman, or a man who has experienced it. Experiencing violence is destructive and threatening to a child or an adult. Work on the consequences in the given person should be embedded in the context of the family of origin, the current family, and the environment in which the person has grown up and lives.

Such a dysfunctional and pathological family system is reinforced by destructive beliefs (myths) existing in the given environment, thus also in the person that comes to the therapy. The myths say that the victim has only one's self to blame; that the perpetrator does not bear any responsibility for their actions or is falsely accused; that the woman and children are to be subordinated to a man, and the man is to be the ruler in the given family; beating and one-off violence is not an abuse and does not leave negative consequences in the life of a child or a grown-up. Those and similar attitudes increase domestic violence in Polish society, decrease the possibility of getting support and protection, and these decreased possibilities reinforce consequences that appear in the person harmed.

Attention should also be paid to the risk factors of domestic violence, the specific ones, which can indicate what particular violence does occur, as well as the non-specific, which only show that some violence is taking place.

When dealing with harmed people it is necessary to be able to recognize what constitutes the pathologic behavior of the active and passive perpetrators in the original or current family, to recognize their mechanisms for hiding or denying the violence and for invoking the feeling of guilt in the victims. The therapist's task during therapy is to model - to build together with the client - a functional reality different from that created by the active and passive perpetrators.

In the family and in the environment as well, the violence is transmitted from generation to generation; so, during therapy it is necessary to take care of two and maybe three generations in a given family. This serves to stop the transmission.

The family also has resources that strengthen a given family and facilitate the introduction of changes. Among them one would count, for instance, flexibility, organization, satisfaction of real needs, coping with decisions and conflicts, and a clear expression of one's feelings and empathy. Parental behaviors demonstrate emotional warmth, support and proximity; stimulate their children emotionally, perceptually and physically; and protect them; in other words, they are responsible and caring. In mutual relations they listen to each other, participate in conversations, give information to each other, feel respect, jointly engage in domestic affairs, co-operate and appreciate each other. Roles, principles and rules are clearly understood and there is no intergenerational mix. And there is plenty of humor within the family. The family feels community and autonomy (Widera-Wysoczańska, 2010).

It is important to properly understand individual, subjective meanings given by a person to the reality they experience. Its symptoms result also from how lived-through experiences are interpreted. Such interpretation appears at the moment violence is experienced; also, recollections of past traumas are interpreted. The events themselves cannot be changed.

In order for the recognition and the change in meaning to occur, methodical recollection and talk about the experienced abuse at the client's own pace are necessary to reveal the secret kept for years and to give real meanings to experienced harm (the father would beat not because he loved nor did he sexually abuse because the child was walking about the house in underwear, but because in this pathologic way by committing a crime he wanted to create his importance. Talking in detail about the facts from the past is particularly important and serves: 1) to stop the secrecy that the perpetrator wants (wanted) to maintain, and disclose the experienced harm, often for the first time in their life; 2) to make contact with reality, a particularly important step for persons who do not react to facts but to their own inner interpretations of the situation they are in - defined by Wallen (1963) as an autistic style; 3) to make the situation from the past and present more realistic in order to get to denied emotions and thoughts and give new meaning to situations from the past (e.g. placing responsibility for harm on the perpetrator and caregiver, who was supposed to protect, and to recognize their responsibility for using abuse and lack of care; 4) to be confronted with the facts, which confrontation enables the start of empathy for oneself (and consequently for one's children), allowing recognition of the harm done, the experience of anger, sadness, regret; 5) to free oneself from dysfunctional family models in order to build new roles in life and an integrated and stable identity.

In persons who have experienced interpersonal trauma, results appear that can assist them over the span of their whole life, often in every sphere: emotional, cognitive, behavioral, somatic, social (family, peers), and spiritual. They can take on different forms, varying with time. With respect to causes of their origin, the consequences the person experiences can be specific (occurring especially after suffering a given, particular form of abuse) and non-specific (indicating that some abuse has been suffered, but what it was is unknown); with respect to the possibility of their recognition: external (behaviors directly visible for an observer, e.g. excitation) and internal (feelings and thoughts non-observable directly on the outside); with respect to their duration and the possibility of making a connection by the client with the harm experienced: immediate responses to the harm, acute and short-term symptoms (symptoms that cease to be visible on the outside after a short time since the harm was experienced) and long-term (chronic; with a slow beginning; when they occur some time after the experienced harm; with remissions; when in a stressful situation the mood aggravation follows), as well as secondary life problems (see Chapter II). Additionally, with respect to their intensity and range of occurrence in a person the following may occur: responses, symptoms, problems and disorders (e.g. complex PTSD), and concurrent disorders. The more time passes since the experienced harm, the more difficult it is for the person to realize where a given life problem and disorder comes from in them.

Violence, when experienced during a person's critical life periods, especially in childhood but in youth as well, influences the development of the human being in a particular way. The earlier a child suffers emotional, physical or sexual violence, the more serious consequences are visible in its life (Erikson, 1980).

Of course, an individual has internalized resources and abilities that enable her (him) to survive childhood abuse and leads them to adulthood in which they realize to a great extent tasks of a grown-up person. Those resources allow them to build a functional future. The symptoms are a way to cope with the harmful experience and with the recollections about it. They make it possible to survive, physically and psychically, in a situation of stress and threat (Briere, 1992; Briere, Scott, 2006). They become destructive when the individual has lost control over them and undergoes the given symptoms in a healthy environment. Then the symptoms hinder response. Each symptom has a positive intent, yet the way the intent is actualized does not always fit the situation the person is in. In extreme situations it may lead to unacceptable behaviors, including domestic violence.

The extent to which the individual remembers their past has great impact on the intensification of the symptoms and ability to heal. Consequences are graver, the earlier the individual experiences the trauma and remembers less (Van der Kolk, 1996a; 1996b). Absence of memories about the violence is connected with its having occurred in the child's life before approximately the third year of life, during, that is, the period of child amnesia (Argenti, Schramm, 2009; Bremner, Scott, et al., 1993; Bremner, Krystal, Southwick, Charney, 1995). In order for the individual to heal faster and more effectively it is important to gain recollection, especially about who the perpetrator was; what happened; in which life period it happened; as well as where it happened. Then the individual may regain control over their life.

Violence is particularly harmful when it comes from a close person, from which one expects security, trust, proximity, and love, namely from parents or caretakers. A great problem arises in a situation where there is dispersed responsibility, when a child taken from their family home has successive caretakers from foster families, who are supposed to provide the child with security, and there the child experiences violence again. The child does not know then who the person most responsible for harm done to them is, and which particular caretaker to be angry at most.

Chronic trauma experienced from a close person disturbs one's ability to trust another person and to feel secure. That is why the role of building a relationship of security between the therapist and the client (a therapeutic alliance) during therapy is emphasized. It serves to rebuild the trust and the sense of security that the harmed person has lost.

As a result of abuse from a close person, a child may build upon their authentic self a fake one, which allows them to adapt to the destructive behaviors of the close person. The child forgets about its own feelings and needs and behaves in accordance with the parent's requirements, blaming itself for the violence experienced. Thus, for the person to be able to heal, they have to detach themselves from their family, be it for some time. Then they have a greater chance to experience feelings that until now they have had to deny (when they remained with the harmful relatives): powerlessness, anger, hate, harm, sadness, loneliness.

It is important to experience sorrow after the loss of a normal childhood. One of the objectives of therapy is for the person to find their authentic self again. Forgiving the close person is not a stage in therapy, but it is additional effect which is not assumed at the beginning of the therapy. Sometimes it is impossible to forgive, since the damages are too great.

In their current life, a person harmed during the childhood behaves like a victim, and at the same time they may, and usually do, act as a perpetrator toward their own relatives: children, partner or parents. The result of this duality is the application of interventions affecting the two intertwined ways of the person's operation. The adult client frees himself/herself in this way from the necessity of keeping in secret the fact that although they suffered harms in childhood, they have also become a perpetrator. That is why therapeutic actions are undertaken from two important perspectives: the grown-up client as a person harmed in childhood, as well as a person that in their adult life hurts other people, their own children in particular.

Table 12-2. Multifacetedness of theoretical perspectives

Theoretical perspectives	Content
Three time perspectives (through life-span)	- past, present and future
Viewing the experienced abuse	- is a truth, not a fantasy - intergenerationally transmitted - its occurrence in a family is affected by destructive beliefs (myths) of the environment
Family of origin and the current one	- functional, dysfunctional, pathologic - mechanisms of the occurrence of various types of abuse - risk factors - resources and possibilities of the family
Dysfunctional, pathologic behaviors of active and passive perpetrators	- mechanisms of abuse - mechanisms of hiding or denying abuse and inducing guilt in victims
Intergenerational transmission of abuse	- transmitting abuse from generation to generation
Subjective interpretation	- individual and subjective meaning given by the individual to the reality experienced by them
Disclosing secrets	- talking about the abuse to disclose the secret, give real meaning to harm
Symptoms and their dynamics	- they appear at the moment an abuse is experienced, e.g. in childhood, and may be present throughout the whole of life - they appear in different forms (external, internal; specific, non-specific; short term and long term; problems, disorders, etc.) - with time they change their form - they are mechanisms of coping with the abuse

	- they become destructive when they appear in a healthy environment and against the individual's will
Dynamics of development influenced by abuse	abuse influences the development of the person during their whole life, in particular when it occurs at critical moments of the life cycle
Resources and capabilities of the individual	- they allow the person to function in spite of the abuse - they allow for development
Memory and ability to remember the traumatic events	The more the person remembers of the experienced abuse, the faster the healing proceeds
Relations with the perpetrator, active and passive	- abuse inflicted by a close person (a parent, a caretaker) is particularly harmful - the lack of support and protection on the part of a close person is particularly harmful - the phenomenon of dispersed responsibility for the abuse inflicted
Authentic and fake self	- Building a fake self upon the authentic one as a result of abuse experienced in childhood - temporary detachment from the family in which abuse has happened
Ambivalence of behaviors: the individual as perpetrator and as victim:	a grown up person as a person abused in childhood and as a person who in adult life abuses other people, in particular their own children

From the above reality that we deal with during psychological interaction, there emerge diagnostic objectives, assumptions about methods applied, and specific ways to conduct the therapy.

Diagnosis of consequences and resources in a person "throughout their life"

When we deal with both grown-ups and children, it is necessary to identify the meaning of their behaviors, the existing symptoms, issues and disorders of early childhood, ever since the time when individuals remember their behaviors up to the point when they come to therapy. The psychotherapist considers how these individuals had functioned in the past (symptoms that occurred in them at that time) and hypothetically foresees how they may function in the future. This provides an opportunity to plan ways of coping with possible problems and methods for fulfilling life plans and objectives. That is why diagnosis of a grown-up person who has come to therapy covers their responses to the harm that has been occurring throughout the whole span of their life. Diagnosis of specific symptoms and risk factors in the family allows the psychotherapist, with a high degree of probability, to understand and find out what kind of abuse the individual had suffered in childhood. This is particularly important when the individual does not remember their past.

Aggravation and changes in symptoms with time should also be considered. The more months or years that have passed since the abuse was experienced, the more complicated the symptoms may have become in the person who comes to the therapy. With the help of the therapist the patient copes with the cumulative consequences of harmful stresses recurring in their life. In the same life period the patient experiences chronic consequences of abuse suffered in childhood by developing secondary life problems as well as consequences resulting from harmful experiences suffered during various life stages in different environments (the family of origin, peer environment, education, professional life, and the current family); respond inappropriately to relatively recent and current stress situations; undergo crises brought about by interaction of childhood harm and those of adult life; and undergo disorders that have emerged as a result of childhood harm (Briere, 2005; Widera-Wysoczańska, 2010).

During diagnosis, however, we do not deal solely with symptoms resulting from the experienced harm. For a person to be able to return to health, it is important to identify that person's inner resources as well as such capabilities as they possess so that they can continue to develop.

A diagnosis of the functional and dysfunctional family of origin and the current family is required. We identify in them forms of abuse and behaviors of the perpetrators'. It is extremely important to identify functional features of those families, their members and mutual relationships in order to indicate an important positive source of strength used by the person in their life (Tab. 12-3).

Table 12-3. Multifacetedness diagnosis of an individual's functioning in the family and environment from the "life-span" perspective.

Groups	Subjects to be diagnosed from a given group
"through time"	1. The individual's past, their present, and planned future - three time perspectives to diagnose the person and the family
Individual - symptoms and resources	1. features and dynamics of the person's development 2. crises 3. resources and capabilities existing in the individual 4. symptoms, problems, and disorders of human a. that take place during the trauma and right after; b. that occur at the recollection of abuses c. that change with the lapse of time 5. ambivalence in the client's behavior, who Is both a victim and a perpetrator
Family of origin and current family as well as the environment	1. functionality of the family of origin and the current one 2. dysfunctionality of the family of origin and the current one 3. risk factors in the family of origin and the current one 4. various abuse mechanisms used in the family 5. pathologic behaviors of active and passive perpetrators in the family 6. intergeneration mechanisms used to intergenerational transmit traumatic events in the given family

The premises regarding the method

Psychotherapeutic methods should be adapted to the theoretical background of the integrative therapy. In them, one takes into account the individual functioning of the abused person (e.g. prohibition to speak, order of silence, submission and loyalty towards the perpetrator, cognitive deformation, blaming herself, and lack of trust) and consideration of one's own capabilities as a therapist. Those methods should be adjusted to the individual needs and emotional and perceptual capabilities of each person and refer to three time periods (working through the life span).

Therapeutic methods used in this approach are based on the assumptions that the abuse has actually happened once the person speaks about it. The abuse is named directly, without reducing its significance, and the perpetrator's behavior is evaluated (Herman, 1992).

It is appreciated that an individual bears consequences as a result of even a one-time abuse, as opposed to denying it or reducing its meaning. Work on the consequences in the given person is embedded in the context of the family of origin, the current family, and the environment in which the person has grown up and lives. The person might not consent to the system that has been ruling in their family so far. The patient is not involved in a therapy that has reconstruction of the family as its priority and that strives to regenerate traditional family roles which, according to some approaches and therapists, can serve as protection against abuse in the family.

First each person must undergo their own individual and group psychotherapy: the victim to build their own strength and a realistic view of the world, and the perpetrator to admit to his guilt and responsibility for his acts, to learn to control his behavior and fantasies (as sexual or physical perpetrator), and not to manipulate victims. Only then, and once the abused person gives fully conscious consent, is it possible to conduct joint therapy for the family members, In the approach presented we do not conduct a systematic therapy in families in which interpersonal, chronic, and complex abuse occurred. The abused child is deprived of a chance to react in accordance with its own experiences, intuitions, and thoughts. So, it is emotionally and perceptually defenseless against the perpetrator sitting next to it and still manipulating (be it with sight) the child and whole family.

In particular, in the initial stages of the therapy it is important to use narrative methods, and not only to work with symbols void of content, which let the person talk about suffered abuse. The process of talking about the abuse allows one to reveal events, sometimes for the first time ever, and "breaks" the mechanism of denying and silence introduced by the perpetrator.

The healing process consists of helping the person to remember and talk about the traumas and the roles, rules, and beliefs in the family from the perspective of an adult in a secure and controlled situation, and of giving new and realistic meaning to those experiences. While helping the person to recollect the past, we use methods that allow the individual to regain control. Thus we avoid methods based on trance, hypnosis or other suggestion.

We propose movement and dance to the patient, instead of methods based on touching the patient's body. If it is to come to "safe touch", we do that, with the patient's consent, at further stages of the therapy, after a detailed investigation of the abuse (eg. sexual) and its consequences, in order for the client to know that they are in control of the situation.

Table 12-4. Recommended and non-recommended approaches in using "life-span" psychotherapy for a person after childhood trauma

Recommended approaches	Not recommended approaches
if the persons talks about abuse experienced in childhood, it means that it occurred; only the perpetrator is responsible for it;	a child or a woman (the victim) is fantasizing or projecting their own needs (e.g. resulting from unsatisfied libidinal needs); when the child talks about abuse (e.g. sexual) and/or says that the child/woman is guilty (e.g. it/she seduced the perpetrator; deserved to be beaten because it/she behaved badly); the person should apologize to the perpetrator
the person does not benefit as a result of the abuse inflicted; on the contrary the violence lowers their potential	acknowledge the reality of the abuse but see it as natural and beneficial to the child (he has grown up to be a decent man because he was beaten)
the person bears consequences even when they experienced a one-time abuse	acknowledge the reality of abuse, but ignore or trivialize the consequences borne by the child/adult
the person might oppose the roles that exist in their family; traditional roles that recognize the man as a ruler, and the woman as a subordinate are risk factors for abuse	strive to rebuild and maintain traditional family roles based on myths

Individual separate therapy for abused persons and for perpetrators of abuse; the perpetrator manipulates the family members be it only with sight, mimics, body - they do not need to say anything	strive to introduce joint, systematic therapy for all members of the family and its system, in which chronic trauma (different types of abuse) has occurred, without consideration of the dynamics of abuse and the perpetrator's manipulative influence on the victim
narrative methods to uncover the secret and to liquidate mechanisms of silence and denial introduced by the perpetrator	apply "contentless" symbolic techniques at the trauma recollection stage
narrative methods in which the person feels conscious control over what and how they are talking when they reveal facts and interpretations from their life	apply hypnosis and other suggestive techniques at the trauma recollection stage
movement, dance without touch; safe touch in further part of the therapy, after the person's life and problems have been diagnosed	apply techniques of working with the body without adequate adjustment to each person and without prior preparation of the person

The methods of psychological help

Therapeutic methods of have been adjusted to the multifaceted and complex abuse phenomenon. Individual and group therapy are most often used. During individual therapy the patient builds a therapeutic alliance with the psychotherapist, diagnosis takes place, and the work on the past begins. Individual therapy is conduced separately to each member of the family.

The group is often the most effective, and is essential for bringing about change. In a group the person works on the past to build both a current and a future life in relationship with the group members and the roles they assume. The patient receives support, realizes they are not alone with their problems, their process of recollection and getting through to the denied feelings is accelerated, they see the problems from the perspective of other members of the group, and transference connected with various family members is initiated.

Crisis intervention is most often applied during the first sessions or in the course of therapy when a crisis arises. It serves to stabilize the current difficult life and psychic situation. Consultation with specialists (e.g. a psychiatrist) is useful, especially at the beginning of therapy in the phase of setting therapeutic priorities. With their participation, it is decided whether a person can take part in the therapy and how it is to proceed.

The person can also take advantage of the therapist's support or of group support; support from colleagues is also important. Owing to it, the person expresses and abreacts feelings connected with the current life situation.

If a woman undergoing therapy demonstrates disturbed attachment to her child, joint therapy sessions of the caregiver with the child based on relational therapy (Widera-Wysoczańska, 2005) are recommended. Its main objectives are processing and then liquidating transference and projection of the caretaker onto the child, changing dysfunctional behaviors and relationships, thus creating new relations. This should not be delayed until the end of the adult's individual therapy, as it often demands immediate intervention. However, it is more effective when the caregiver has already participated in their own therapy for some time, and they have decreased the degree of transference from their own parents or partner to the child (for example, it is difficult for a mother to accept her own son if she sees in him the perpetrator because she had been molested by her father).

In the last integration phase, after completing the individual therapy of the particular family members, a joint family therapeutic session may take place, if the harmed person so wishes. The perpetrator is seldom is involved in coming to such a decision: When making this decision one must consider whether the perpetrator has also been treated and whether changes in him are evident. A situation like this, however, is not very likely and seldom occurs.

Thematic developmental groups are suggested in the last phase of the therapy. The participants, for example, develop their upbringing, partner, and assertive skills, or set goals and plan how they can be reached.

The strategies and techniques

The selection of techniques depends on the client's needs, the kind of symptoms, the form of abuse experienced, the stage of the therapy, and goals which are to be realized. They should also be adjusted to the level at which changes are to be implemented, that is, to the environment, the person's behavior, values, and beliefs, or to the level of identity (Dilts

Robert, after: McDermott, Jago, 2006). The therapist must be flexible in applying strategies and technique with various therapeutic approaches.

During the particular stages, the techniques from various approaches are usually employed: humanistic, psychodynamic, relational, behavioral-cognitive, stress coping, experimental/cathartic, metaphoric including Ericksonian and NLP, or expressive techniques and psychodrama. The techniques employed are:

- narrative: retrospective and exploratory
- insight directed
- directed towards abreaction and processing of emotions
- changing cognitive distortions and beliefs
- confrontation directed
- building relationships with people
- teaching stress coping
- teaching new behaviors
- directed towards bringing forth resources and development

Duration

Because of the chronic, complex, and interfamily nature of abuse, its impact on the development of the personality and the strength and intensity of the symptoms, this therapy is long-term. It is a therapy directed towards a goal. This means that its duration is determined by the person who has goals to realize. Some people feel better when they have a defined timeframe. This therapy may last from about one to seven years, most often about three years. The frequency of sessions depends on the stage of the therapy and its character. At first, individual sessions take place once a week and not more often. The person has to have time to introduce changes in their daily life: recollection, building new relations with people, creating boundaries, and regaining strength and control over the emotional and cognitive sphere. Sessions take place more often in an acute crisis. During the final stages, individual sessions may take place every two weeks, once a month, or less often. The rule is to gradually decrease the number of sessions.

During these sessions the therapist accompanies the client in a gradual and accelerated development, monitoring to assure that there is maturation under secure conditions. The person gradually becomes independent of the therapist, just as a maturing child does from its parents. The therapist, just as a healthy parent, must create conditions of security so that the client can go out into the world independently and safely.

Some people do not consent to reaching back into the past and want to deal with specific, individual symptoms or problems in their current life. Then one applies a short-term therapy (Table 12-5).

Table 12-5. Duration of the psychotherapy for a person after childhood abuse

Duration	Description
Long-term (due to the nature of chronic and complex trauma and interfamily abuse)	- work on causes and consequences - duration determined by goals which the person wants to realize - mean duration of the main stages is about three years - the frequency of sessions decreases during therapy
Short-term	when the person wants to deal with specific problems and has not decided to work on their life history

The stages of integrative therapy

Integrative therapy consists of strategies divided with respect to its process (cf.: Briere, 1988; Courtois, 1998; Pearlman, 1998, Salter, 1988; 2003; Widera-Wysoczańska, 2007) and with respect to its form and goals intended.

The stages of "life-span" therapy with respect to the process

The stages of process of the "life-span" integrated therapy follow the changes that clients introduce into their own lives. Those include (Tab 12-6) identification, diagnosis, stabilization and setting priorities; disclosure and recollection; processing the post-traumatic consequences; and integration of the past, present and future. These stages include phenomena that indicate the multithreaded nature of the processes and themes used in healing the person.

During the first stage - identification, diagnosis, stabilization and setting priorities - diagnoses are made of the person, family and the environment in which the person currently lives. On this basis the priorities of the treatment are set. The priority tasks include situations in which the person is currently experiencing abuse from a parent or partner, has suicidal tendencies, has depression which makes normal functioning impossible, abuses alcohol or drugs, suffers from eating disorders (bulimia, anorexia) and troubling somatic complaints, is emotionally, physically, or sexually aggressive (towards their children or partner), or shows psychotic symptoms. At an appropriate time and while under observation by proper specialists, all these persons may return to a therapy involving the impact of the past on their current lives.

Another stabilizing and security-providing action is establishing therapeutic contact as well as building a safe therapist-patient relationship. In order to start transferring the effects of therapy from the office to the patient's current life at this stage, the patient is to establish contact with people who support them, from outside the family of origin and the current one. Clients also recognize in themselves their own resources needed to cope with the current situation (they are strong because they have survived, because, after all, they work, bring up children, have come to therapy, etc.).

The second stage - disclosure and recollection (memory management) - that runs almost parallel to the first and third stages, concerns gradual recollection from the past (e.g. the family of origin or school) of the facts about the abuse (what, who, where, when and how; relations, principles, roles, mechanisms and myths). This is done in order to disclose the secret concerning abuse and stopping the isolation, recognizing facts and giving them more realistic meanings (work with cognitive distortions), and getting through to denied emotions by "coming in contact" with facts. Disclosure does not mean solving the problems, but it is an initial stage of the healing process from childhood trauma, making the experienced abuse real and providing a basis for further diagnosis of the person.

During the third stage - processing the post-traumatic consequences - the patient deals with symptoms that have resulted from the abuse being experienced within the family, recognizes and abreacts feelings (e.g. guilt, shame, anger, regret, sadness), identifies and modifies beliefs that are cognitive distortions, copes with the loyalty to perpetrators, and confronts from the position of an adult the main offender and other family members who have not protected and supported them when they were abused. The expected result is gaining control and power.

Eventually the patient, becoming aware of and accepting the positive aspects of one's own past, learns from the trauma how to seek constructive help from others and how to avoid destruction; frees herself/himself from suppressed feelings and from illusions of the "loving family" (“bursting the soap bubble”) and builds a realistic view of the family of origin, which allow the person to build authentic and secure relationships. When the clients become aware of and accept the positive aspects of their own past and the parents' behavior, they may realize that besides the difficult moments in their lives there have been good ones as well, which gives them force to live.

In parallel to these processes, psychological help is delivered to the patient's children who also may have suffered abuse and need help. The person is building a new parent-child relationship. They need to examine their understanding of the process of child abuse, the consequences for the child and other members of the family and the situation after the disclosure, as well as the reactions of the caregiver to the disclosure. The caregiver must start learning new behaviors towards the child. The parent must analyze the denial concerning the abuse practiced by themselves, the child, the perpetrator, and the environment. The person must take responsibility for the child's safety, learn to recognize and react to the perpetrator's manipulation and effectively support the child and help the child cope with the consequences. At the same time the caregiver must deal with building a safe home, setting boundaries (especially with sexual abuse) such that the child's intimacy is not infringed upon, abiding by stables rules, and so on.

At this stage of the therapy many patients recognize their own abusive behavior towards other people. Some of the persons had already revealed inflicting emotional or physical abuse and neglect before as well as transgressing their child's intimate boundaries. They were, however, unable to identify with this behavior and take conscious (and emotional) responsibility for it. Usually they are prepared to recognize and admit their own abusive behaviors against others, learn to accept responsibility for having hurt the children and partners, and learn to hear from those close to them about their behavior as an offender. Some of the persons (both women and men) admit to sexual abuse in their adult life of their own or somebody else's child, as well as in their childhood and youth - of a sibling or a peer. The goal of this stage is to cope with being a perpetrator of emotional, physical, and sexual violence of one's own children, partner, or parents: stopping destructive and criminal behaviors, accepting responsibility for one's own actions, and building empathy. Our experience shows that persons, when they have first dealt with abuses they experienced in their own childhood, have better prospects in controlling their own behaviors as perpetrators.

The fourth stage - integration of the past, present and future (new behaviors, goals, and plans) - serves to build the present and future life. The person should bring about changes in their current life (leave the toxic home, find work, build relationships, and get more education). Early identification in oneself as a perpetrator of violence against others makes it possible to stop many destructive behaviors, and this facilitates building a bond between parent and child, building a bond with the partner, as well as improving interpersonal, assertive, upbringing and partner skills. The person should build more realistic expectations of others and themselves solve current life problems concerning relationships, and set boundaries, rules, roles, and values in different areas of life. The person is also prepared to plan their life, and undertake important decisions that build up their current and future life.

Table 12-6. The stages of "life-span" integrative therapy with respect to the process

The stages of integrative therapy	With reference to the processes
I. Identification and stabilization	- diagnosis of the person and identification of their environment - treatment priorities and contact with specialists - stabilization and security (building a mature therapist-patient relationship, "contract" with supportive persons)

II. Disclosure and "recollection"	- organizing the memory: what, where, when, how
	- facts and particulars concerning:
	    - coming from a dysfunctional family (rules, roles, mechanisms, myths)
	    - the abuse experienced and
	    - recalling symptoms from childhood to adulthood (if people do not remember the traumatic events exactly, or they are afraid they are only imagined; recalling symptoms confirms the reality of the trauma)

III. "Processing" post-traumatic consequences	- regarding the dysfunctional family and experienced abuse - identifying and abreacting emotions - identifying and changing beliefs (distortions) - confronting the main perpetrator and other family members - becoming aware of and accepting the positive aspects of one's own past and the parents'/caregivers' behavior - recognizing one's own abusive behavior towards other people
IV. Integration of the past, present, and future	- identifying oneself as a perpetrator of abuse of one's own children, partner, parents, and other people and changes in behavior - building child-parent attachment - building partner attachment - building and improving skills in: - interpersonal relations - assertiveness - upbringing - partnership - planning and realizing goals and making decisions

The stages of the integrated psychotherapy with regard to structure

Integrative psychotherapy covers many forms of work with the patient which, on the basis of individual problems to be solved that were revealing themselves during the work, have gradually completed and filled up its structure. Inside these forms the processes described above occur. In this way a multifaceted model of psychotherapy has originated (tab. 12-7).

The structure has been divided into five stages ("classes"). In order to participate in the next stage, the client usually should have completed the preceding one.

Table 12-7. The forms of the integrated psychotherapy

Stage	Sequence of the forms of the therapy	Method
I stage	1. "preparatory" sessions	individual
	2. "basic" for persons from dysfunctional families and for those who experienced abuse	group (+individual)
	3. parent-child attachment	individual
	4. the couple's relationship	individual
II stage	5. persons who experienced sexual abuse or persons who experienced abuse in the family	group (+individual) group (+individual)
III stage	6. for perpetrators or for parents who support children	group (+individual) individual or group
IV stage	7. developmental-"thematic"	group
	8. therapeutic sessions	individual
V stage	9. incidental crises session	individual

It begins with several individual "preparatory" sessions that are to prepare the person for group therapy. During these sessions the person and their environment are diagnosed, the goals of the therapy and indicators of achieving these goals are set, priorities and risk factors are diagnosed, and supportive persons are identified. During these sessions the patient fills in questionnaires prepared specially for this integrative therapy. They fill them in again at the completion of every stage.

Another form of work is "basic" group therapy that, because of the patients' problems, is called "therapy for persons from dysfunctional families and who experienced abuse". During this group process the patient copes with the consequences of growing up in a dysfunctional family, discloses the abuse in front of the therapy group, recognizes the causes of current problems, gains courage to leave home, and owing to relationships in the group learns to build mature relationships and to introduce changes in her/his current life.

At the same time, if necessary, the third form of "patient-child attachment" therapy might be introduced. It has as objectives the recognition of the abuse inflicted by caretakers upon the child, the construction of an attachment with the child based on trust and security, and the learning of ways to protect the child. At a later (final) stage of group therapy, the construction of a partner relationship occurs, in the form of individual meetings. The third and fourth forms of psychotherapy might be continued during the stages that follow.

The second stage of the therapy takes care of women who experienced sexual abuse. It is focused on healing the traumas of sexual abuse from childhood and other stages of life, coping with crises, setting goals for the future, and building mother-child and partner relationships. Optionally, if the person has not experienced sexual abuse, they may take part in heterogeneous group therapy for persons who did experience abuse in the family.

Another, third stage of the psychotherapeutic work is group therapy for perpetrator-persons abused in childhood who during preceding stages of therapy recognized a perpetrator in themselves (recognized behavior typical of abusive perpetrators) of emotional, physical, or sexual abuse of their own children, partners, and parents. In the stage concerning perpetrator recognition in oneself, the following special phases of healing appear: recognition of one's own behavior as an offender, preventing destructive behaviors, investigating which toxic rules of the dysfunctional family and incest in childhood have been transferred into adult life, learning to accept responsibility for inflicting violence against children and parents, learning empathy and hearing from close ones about one's behavior as an offender, and building new constructive relationships, rules, roles, boundaries and ways of behavior.

There is also a group for persons, mostly mothers, who have a problem with supporting and protecting their own child from abuse (mainly sexual) inflicted by other people.

The fourth stage consists of participation in developmental thematic groups during which people develop social skills, assertiveness, rearing skills, good marital relations, and learn to plan for the future and cope with stress. Some persons continue the therapy during individual sessions.

The therapeutic process ends with incidental individual sessions when the person needs support during serious crises and would like to obtain help in solving current life problems.

Methods for monitoring the effectiveness of the therapy

During initial individual sessions, the patient fills in questionnaires specially prepared for the integrative therapy described. They fill them in again on the completion of each stage of the treatment. These questionnaires allow one to study the effectiveness of the therapy conducted to that point, and indicate further issues to be resolved and objectives to be realized.

Methods have been developed (Widera-Wysoczańska, 2010) for studying 1) the motive and goals of the person participating in the therapy, 2) symptoms that occur in the person from childhood until the time they enter therapy, 3) the situation in the family of origin, in the current one, and abuse experienced in life, and 4) a review of the therapy and planning further actions with the end result of healing the individual.

In the first group, an interview is found at the beginning of the therapy to examine the current life situation of the patient and their motivation and objectives for undergoing treatment. Symptoms are identified with the help of a questionnaire, the Questionnaire of Somatic Disorders (QSD), to examine health problems that occur at different periods of life and concern all somatic systems. In addition we use DES - II (*Dissociative Experiences Scale*, by Carlson and Putnam, Putnam, 1997) to examine the kind of dissociation, and selected questionnaires to identify possible personality disorders and the psychical condition of the individual. In order to identify kinds of sexual abuse experienced, I have created structured questionnaires "Intimate Situations of Women" (ISW) and "Intimate Situations of Men" (ISM) to identify the type of sexual/physical abuse suffered and of addictions at various periods in the person's life; I also use the Domestic Abuse Form (DAF) as well as "Retrospective Perception of Parent's Behaviors" (RPPB, Cronbach's alpha = 0.94) that shows subjective perceptions of the father's and mother's behavior in the childhood of the individual examined (Widera-Wysoczańska, 2010, 2010a). With the help of a qualitative form, we examine the relation with the partner and the childhood bonds with mother and father that influence this relation. On completion, patients fill in "an interview at the end of therapy", in which they evaluate the extent and the quality of their changes in different spheres of life and plan further a course of action to increase their quality of life.

Traps in the healing process

In the healing process there are crises that result from rules set up in childhood in a dysfunctional family. Both the patient who inflicts violence and the one who does not protect the child behave in such a way that calls into question the child's faith in its safety and in its understanding of the sense and goodness of this world. When choosing the preferred psychotherapeutic method, the therapist should consider the impact that this harmful pashas had on the patient.

Issues on the part of the person being healed

Problems occur when an adult does not remember much from the past or does not want to access memories. Yet, sleeping daemons from the past require an insight into one's past. The individual might be forbidden to speak and ordered to maintain secrecy and silence; thus their experiences are ignored, and any awareness of their own reality is distorted by pretending that nothing happened.

A threat to the healing process might be the willingness of our patient to take care of their family, not of themselves. This might be an escape from dealing with their own difficulties. And yet, the patient should realize that they will not change their parents and that their healing does not depend upon the healthy condition of their family.

Healing is connected with no longer protecting the perpetrator, and by a person dependent on them. However, accusations then arise from family members of the abused child's cold, distanced, cruel and egoistic behaviors. This reinforces in the patient a feeling of disloyalty to the parents and triggers a feeling of guilt towards them. Such persons believe that they are guilty of and responsible for everything, and that they must be ashamed (but the perpetrator is without guilt), and that they are subordinate to, and forced into destructive loyalty to, the perpetrator.

Another threat is the tendency to attribute all of life's problems to the family or to attribute none. Such an abused child does not want to realize that something bad is happening to it. This person is controlled in such a way that they have lost all sense of their own power, inner control and value. Since they have been repeatedly betrayed, first by the perpetrator, then by the caregiver, who did not react to beatings or sexual abuse, and by other family members, and by strangers in the environment (teachers, trainers), they display distorted trust in the most important persons, and therefore in all others. We meet a patient who does not accept closeness, feels self-hatred, and has no empathy for themselves (this results in a lack of empathy for others and their own children), and who shows aggression inappropriate to the situation and often employs transferred aggression. In them, particularly strong transference feelings toward the therapist occur, in whom they may see the perpetrator, the bad parent, or the good parent, and from whom they may demand emotional or actual "adoption" and with whom they experience accelerated maturity. An increased feeling of loneliness is also a threat.

During the healing process, moments of bad mood occur. When fear and pain caused by increasing awareness of life's situation dominate feelings that go together with healing, then anxiety appears. The client wants one's work over oneself finished quickly. In reality this anxiety should be an indication that problems need to be resolved. Another threat to development is "resting on one's laurels" after having made basic changes in oneself and having set goals for the future. To heal oneself, it is necessary to be continually engaged in making changes permanent (Table 12-8).

Table 12-8. Traps appearing in the client during "life-span" psychotherapy

- prohibition to speak
- cognitive distortion
- guilt and misplaced responsibility
- loyalty to the perpetrator
- lack of inner control, low sense of self-esteem
- loss of trust
- repeated betrayal
- resentment for loss
- hate and lack of self-empathy
-transferred aggression
- transference
- "resting on one's laurel"

Threats on the part of the therapist

All of these special dynamic processes impact the therapist and the therapeutic process. They demand particular attention from the therapist and require effective management of counter-transference. I have carried out research on counter-transference among 60 women therapists who do therapy with persons after abuse: both victims and perpetrators (Widera-Wysoczańska, 2010). Among other things, it follows from that research that the therapist may not wish to become involved in these problems because they cannot cope with the horror of what they hear. They may pretend there is no problem; they avoid it by not identifying the symptoms in the client, not taking up the subject of abuse or asking difficult questions about facts concerning violence, sexual or physical ("it's better not to hear it, because what to do with it then?"). They do not react to the perpetrator's criminal behavior; they turn themselves off and do not hear stories about events the perpetrator is describing, they do not directly call the perpetrator's criminality a crime, and do not confront the perpetrator with the wrong-doings they have committed. When the patient talks about behaviors similar to those that the therapist had experienced previously, the therapist vindicates the patient and sets lower requirements for the patient. When, for instance, the therapist gives slaps the client might consider them permissible. The therapist might be ironic and appraise the patient generally, not the patient's particular sense of having been abused. They may feel power over the patient via the directive nature of therapeutic work and expect quick improvement and change; if not quick enough, they may believe that the patient is "good for nothing" and "is to go away". They may treat the patient condescendingly and feel even hostility towards the patient. They withdraw from the relation, often because of fear and a feeling of powerlessness. At the same time, interestingly, they have a tendency to absolve the client from what she/he has done. They easily lose motivation to deal with such a client and avoid any contact with them.

The therapist may feel guilty that his client experienced childhood abuse and is still experiencing it or he may blame the client that she deserved the abuse ("why did she walk around in a short skirt?"); especially male therapists may become furious when they hear about the sexual abuse of a child.

Some therapists may excessively focus on sexual details, if the client was sexually abused; others may seduce the client and have sexual intercourse with them. The feeling of threat emerges in them as it does with a perpetrator: They panic, feeling powerless and helpless. In such a state they allow the perpetrator manipulate them by using, for instance, aggression and complaints or "being nice" to dictate terms to the therapist and control the course and rules of the meetings. In a similar manner, however, the victim may also manipulate the professional by displaying mechanisms of powerlessness. Then the therapist is ready to withdraw from the relationship and to avoid working with a client like that. Or, again inappropriately, they may assume responsibility for the patient - whether victim or perpetrator - in undertaking actions that should serve healing, as in taking care of life matters for the patient (eg. guessing their states, when the patient does not access them by themselves; giving advice about how to behave; writing communications to the court; taking them in for a night at the therapist's home, finding an apartment for them). In this way the therapist reinforces the sense of powerlessness in the patient.

So the therapist has difficulty in keeping the boundary between themselves and the client. It also happens that the therapist, moved by the story of the client - the perpetrator or the victim of domestic violence -, may recount situations from their own life and deal with themselves, not the client (Table 12-9).

All these reactions result in repeated victimization of the client during the therapeutic relationship.

Table 12-9. Threats to the client on the part of the therapist in "life-span" psychotherapy

- processes appearing in the therapist's own life when in contact with the client - does not wish to become involved in these problems - cannot cope with the horror - pretends there is no problem - avoids diagnosis - does not ask difficult questions about facts - does not react to the perpetrator's criminal behavior as described by the wrongdoer - does not name directly the perpetrator's criminal behavior and does not confront them with the crimes they committed - therapist vindicates the perpetrator's behaviors - is ironic and appraises the patient, not their behavior - feels power over the patient - expects fast improvement - absolves the perpetrator of what the perpetrator has done - easily loses motivation to take care of the patient - demonstrates fury at the perpetrators - feels guilty that they themselves did not experience abuse - blames the victim that it was her fault - questions inordinately about sexual details - seduces and has intercourse with the client - withdraws from a relationship with the patient, often out of fear and a feeling of powerlessness - feels threatened in the relationship with the perpetrator - is manipulated by the victim - is manipulated by the perpetrator - therapist has trouble maintaining the border-line between the herself/himself and the client - therapist recounts their own life situations

What the professional should know

To summarize, doing psychotherapy with individuals who have experienced childhood traumas requires knowledge about many phenomena and processes. To cure such a person, one must have special knowledge about, for instance: 1) types of abuse and trauma, 2) mechanisms and dynamics of abuse in the family, 3) factors concerning intergenerational transmission of violence in the family and environment, 4) consequences which appear throughout the person's life, 5) memory processes, 6) neurological processes in the brain and their influence on changes or absence of changes, 7) diagnosis of a person and their family with respect to resources and troubles, 8) factors leading up to a traumatic event, 9) factors conducive to quick healing, 10) how the person is functioning throughout therapy, and 11) methods of psychological effect adjusted to age and the person's character traits of as well as to their goals and stage of the therapy. In-depth knowledge by the psychotherapist about oneself and their own reactions is also necessary.

CHAPTER THIRTEEN

THE PSYCHOTHERAPY OF ALCOHOLICS - PERPETRATORS OF DOMESTIC VIOLENCE

DOROTA DYJAKON

The article presents the psychotherapy of alcoholics - perpetrators of domestic violence as a proposal which enriches the therapeutic offer for addicted persons. It also turns attention to the special nature of problems which arise in an alcoholic family in relation to using violence by addicted persons not only in an active phase of the disease but also after starting treatment. It also points out violence as a vital element impeding the healing process of an alcoholic family and constituting the source of disturbances related to experiencing chronic trauma.

Addiction to alcohol and reconvalescence in alcoholism

According to diagnostic criteria of The International Statistical Classification of Diseases and Related Health Problems (ICD-10) the addiction to alcohol is defined as an occurrence of at least three of the following symptoms, in the period of at least one month or, during the previous year, in a few periods shorter than one month:

1. Strong thirst or feeling of compulsion to drink ("craving for alcohol").
2. Impairment of abilities to control behavior related to drinking (impairment of abilities to restrain from drinking, difficulties with quitting alcohol, difficulties in limiting the amount of drinking alcohol).
3. Physiologic symptoms of abstinence syndrome in the act of restraining or quitting drinking (tremor, arterial hypertension, nausea, vomiting, diarrhoea, insomnia, anxiety, and in extreme situations tremor delirium) or using alcohol in order to free oneself from abstinence syndromes.

4. Changed (most often increased) toleration for alcohol, a need to drink larger doses in order to achieve the desired effect.
5. Concentration of life on drinking, neglecting one's interests and responsibilities.
6. Persistent drinking of alcohol despite obvious evidence of harmful consequences of drinking.

These criteria indicate the physiologic and psychological nature of addiction which is based on increased alcohol tolerance, the physiologic consequences of quitting alcohol and progressive life adjustments in drinking alcohol. Its chronic and progressive nature is crucial, too, and thereby there is no possibility for its complete cure but only inhibiting an increasing of its symptoms and dangers to health related to it.

In the light of modern knowledge, addiction to alcohol is a multifactorial disease, that is, a bio-psycho-social (Mellibruda, 1997) damaging the functioning of a human being in somatic, psychological, social and spiritual spheres. The treatment model for this disease, then, must be adjusted to the manner of its perception.

An analysis of the process of reconvalescence (cf. Brown, 1990; Gorski, Miller, 1991; Brown, Lewis, 1999) indicates that addiction is a state which causes an obsessive urge to take a given substance (alcohol, drugs, painkillers or hallucinogens) by an addicted person despite negative consequences experienced by him / her. However, reconvalescence is a developmental process requiring complete and strict abstinence in which several stages are identified. During this process important changes appear not only in the functioning of an addicted person but also in family relations. In the period preceding treatment, an alcoholic experiences numerous negative consequences of drinking thanks to which the addicted person realizes that he / she is not able to control drinking alcohol. If the process proceeds successfully, in the end an alcoholic will admit defeat and undergo treatment. Then, the transition phase occurs, connected with experiencing abstinence syndrome (a generalized state of hyperactivity, anxiety, irritability, insomnia, lack of appetite, tachycardia, and tremors) and remission of the most severe symptoms of chronic abstinence syndrome (inability to think clearly, problems with memory, emotional hyperactivity or apathy, sleep disorders, problems with physical coordination, and susceptibility to stress) and slowly begins to regain control over thinking processes, emotions, memory, and ability to behave and judge realistically. This stage mainly hinders the psychological, physical and social destruction of an addicted person constituting the basis to gain “the identity of an alcoholic”.

The next important moment is to learn to live without drugs and alcohol. It is also the phase of compensating for the damages created in the physical, psychological and social sphere caused by addiction. The important element of this process refers to gaining knowledge about addiction not only by the family but also by the patient, which allows one to further understand and accept addiction, estimate the stage of progress of addiction and co-addiction, and get to know personal difficulties in life in order to get started solving life problems. This is also a period of intensive work over problems related to harm made to other people. Further process of reconvalescence leads to achieving a balance in life and developing a normal, based-on-soberness style of life by the alcoholic. The larger sphere of an alcoholic's consciousness occupies work and family. The authors pinpoint that concentration on addiction and an adjusted style of life is essential even when a person has already been a long-term abstainer. In the process of treatment, emphasis should be put on professional, social activity (especially on contacts with family and friends), one's own development, relaxation, sport, being on a special diet and learning how to cope with stress as protection against "substitute addictions" (for example excessive coffee drinking, sex, pornography, and gorging).

The further period of reconvalescence is characterized by work of the addicted person to consolidate changes in identity and behavior. The basic element of this process refers to the development of adequate self-esteem, developing abilities to come into close contact with people, and building a happy and productive life. Also in this phase addicted people are starting to work on other emotional problems that result, for example, from living in an alcoholic family or a family in which there is another dysfunction. The result of this work will be liberation from psychological trauma experienced in childhood, erroneous beliefs about oneself and the surrounding world, as well as creating an adequate image of oneself and one's system of values.

Keeping soberness is the continuation of the process of reconvalescence. The aim of this phase is to realize that addiction is a chronic and incurable disease; therefore this process can never be completed. The main problem in this period is to cope with relapses and to perfect abilities in recognizing warning signs which are aimed at solving problems occurring in life.

Violence in alcoholism

In this study violence is defined as

> all non-accidental acts infringing personal freedom of an individual, which contribute to physical or psychological harm of another human being and which go beyond social norms of mutual human relations (Pospiszyl, 1999, p. 16).

The advantage of this definition refers to avoidance of focusing attention on proving the intention of a person using violence but the centre of gravity rests rather with the damages which these actions may cause. Considering this definition, not only physical violence is the subject of the analysis but every action which does harm to a victim.

Alcoholism is inherently connected with violence. According to statistics, up to 87% of murderers drink alcohol, and over 50% of all penal acts are connected with using alcohol or other psychoactive substances (Niehoff, 2001). Obviously an offender does not have to be always under the influence of alcohol to commit crime. In many situations the lack of alcohol or the means for getting alcohol can be the motive for committing punishable offences.

Very similar in numbers are statistics referring to domestic violence, where an evident contribution of alcohol is visible. Seven out of nine examined occurrences of domestic violence were committed under the influence of alcohol (Hotaling and Sugarman, 1986 after Herzberger, 2002). It was also noted that men abusing alcohol or drugs more often use violence than men without addiction problems. The influence of alcohol on mistreating children plays an equally vital role. Parents abusing alcohol more often neglect their children, harming them emotionally and physically.

Violence in an alcoholic family is also a major problem in Poland. According to police statistics, about 83% of perpetrators of domestic violence are under the influence of alcohol (the number of perpetrators of domestic violence under the influence of alcohol totaled 61 991 in 2008, and the total number of perpetrators of domestic violence totaled 86 568 in 2008)[1]. Therefore, violence in an alcoholic family seems to be quite an obvious problem; however, as the statistics indicate, it is mainly associated with an active phase of the disease (i.e. during the period of abusing alcohol). Then, an alcoholic is seen as a person who neglects family, is aggressive, indifferent, and for whom the most important thing is to get alcohol. Obviously this is a stereotype which comes out in our common view on the person addicted to alcohol. The reality of family where violence appears, however, tends to be more complex and less clear for an ordinary witness. It proves that not only in the active phase of alcoholism does a family experience violence but such a behavior is also present after starting treatment, that is, during the process of reconvalescence, although it is less obvious. There are two reasons for domestic violence. The first results from mental disorders experienced by an addicted person even before turning to drink, and which later contribute to reaching for psychoactive substances including alcohol. Application of alcohol playing the role of "medicine" for psychological troubles causes expansion of problems occurring as a consequence of addiction. Such treatment of the problem is mainly raised by psychoanalytic and neo-psychoanalytic concepts which place disorders in personality development leading to addiction at the centre of attention (cf. Cierpiałkowska, 2000, 2008) and personality concepts (Sher, Trull, Bartholow, Vieth, 2003). Presentation of these ideas in an over-simplified form is to show that not only alcohol has an influence on the behavior of an alcoholic, but also the fact that the addicted person struggles with a variety of other problems before he / she becomes addicted and that these problems do not disappear after stopping drinking that is in the course of treatment. Numerous studies on domestic violence indicate that personality disorders and specific personality constructors are treated as one of the more important factors (cf. Hamberger, Hastings, 1986; Baron, Richardson, 1994; Dutton 1998,). The second reason for violence arises from the process of addiction to alcohol itself and its influence on human behavior in the course of which degradation of higher feelings, values, principles and norms, emotional regulation disorders and development and functioning of specific personality mechanisms takes place (Mellibruda, 1999). Some of the experts on the problem distinguish violence performed by alcoholics as specific for addiction. Denzin (1988, 2007) distinguishes five types of violence characteristic of alcoholism, namely violence which is emotional playful, spurious and/or accidental, real, and paradoxical. He claims that violence which the family experiences from the alcoholic results from his / her “divided self”, which is described as “me sober" and “me under the influence of alcohol”. The experience of such a division causes alcoholics to have their inner world divided into two opposite existences: subjective self and the other self. This "split life" is a contradiction of the self, causing deep inner dissonance in the structure of identity. Using alcohol deepens this division leading also to an emotional split of "myself" (self). The subjective self, as happens also with the other self, is overcome by negative emotions including anger, fear, disgust for oneself, complaining, hatred for oneself, resentment, despair, suffering, remorse, guilt and shame. What happens in the life of an alcoholic is separated from an alcoholic-deformed awareness of a suffering, sick body and its inside. Possibilities for appropriately assessing a situation are restricted to a large extent. His / her alcoholic "proud self" drives negative emotions towards other people. The explanation of this phenomenon lies in perceiving the trap, which functions in the form of an inner vicious circle, and which deepens the discrepancies between alcoholic and non-alcoholic behavior. The alcoholic is starting to be lost in experiencing diametrically different emotions connected with contacts with other people. If this process is not stopped by treatment, it will change into self-destruction. This process also affects the development of domestic violence. Violence in an alcoholic family takes the same forms as in families without any alcoholic problems. It includes physical, verbal and sexual violence which appears occasionally or regularly. Its scope covers such extreme situations as sexual abuse of children, threats to family members with a weapon (for example, a knife, axe or gun), and it can involve beatings, driving under the influence of alcohol and murder.

The pattern of violent behavior used by alcoholics can be very diverse, and can be further established and expanded while drinking. To a large extent it depends on such individual characteristics as personality disorders, stable or changing moods, whether an alcoholic is under the influence of alcohol or is sober, what his / her emotional stability is, predictability or unpredictability of behavior, intentionality or non-intentionality of actions, and dominant feelings towards others such as politeness or cruelty, harshness and avoiding contacts, withdrawal, amicability, hostility and anger. Also, the stage of advancement of the alcoholic disease is firmly related to changes in his / her emotional sphere. Taking into consideration the two approaches, it can be expected that after quitting alcohol, in the course of treatment, patterns of behaviors do not change and alcoholics will still use violence (Dyjakon, 2005, 2007, 2010).

Treatment of addiction

In accordance with the nature of the alcohol disease, psychotherapy of addicted persons requires both medical treatment and psychotherapy. Making some far-reaching generalization it can be said that the treatment program for addicted people is conducted in three stages (Cierpiakowska, 2000): 1) a stationary or ambulatory individual treatment program, including detoxification; 2) group psychotherapy; 3) a continuation of the treatment in support groups e.g. AA. Group psychotherapy in most cases, in Cierpiałkowska's opinion (2000), is of a behavioral-cognitive or eclectic character including relevant ideas of various theoretical approaches. By synthesizing various approaches to the therapy, the following areas can be distinguished: 1) maintaining abstinence and gaining a new identity by a person addicted; 2) handling somatic and psychic disorders caused by alcohol misuse; 3) handling stress and difficult situations; 4) redressing past harms caused by drinking in personal and social (especially family) life; 5) solving one's interpersonal and intra-psychic problems (cf. Brown, 1992; Mellibruda, Sobolewska, Cierpiałkowska, 2000). It seems significant that problems connected with an alcoholic's application of violence are an important element of therapy offered to alcoholics.

Psychotherapy of alcoholics as the perpetrators of domestic violence

Among various therapy proposals applied as therapy proposals for problems with domestic violence (Dutton, 2003), we can divide those which are based on psychoanalytical theory, on relationship and attachment, and on systematic and behavioral cognitive theories. Each of them indicates a different aspect of human functioning and differently interprets problems appearing in his or her life, especially the problems leading to acts of violence.

Theoretical assumptions of the psychotherapy of alcoholics as perpetrators of domestic violence

In the therapy which I developed, I took into consideration both the strategic-structural approach developed by Jerzy Mellibrudy's team (1999) in the treatment of alcohol-addicted persons (assumptions of behavioral and cognitive therapy applied in the therapy for perpetrators of domestic violence), and principles of rational-emotive theory by Ellis (1999).

Fundamental theoretical assumptions

Addicted people participating in the Psychotherapy of Perpetrators of Domestic Violence (PPDV)

1. They continue to abstain from psycho-active agents.
2. In the course of detox therapy, they have obtained basic knowledge and insight into problems resulting from their addiction to alcohol (in the emotional, physical, social and spiritual spheres).
3. They have got essential awareness of violence affected by them towards family members.
4. They are capable of taking responsibility for their actions in both the past and the present.
5. The purpose of participation in PPDV is to satisfy incurred injustice and to restrict the application of violent behaviors in their current life.

People who undertook basic addiction therapy and stayed from eight to 14 weeks free of alcohol took part in the psychotherapy. The therapeutic group was closed and consisted of 10 -12 people at a time. Duration of the therapy - 60 hours of group therapy. The meetings were held once a week for four hours (16 meetings). The meetings took 16 weeks overall. The participants were alcohol-addicted men after basic addiction therapy in the form of ambulatory treatment. The aim of the psychotherapy conducted was 1) changes of identity (increase integrity, continuity, and identification within the family as a point of reference); 2) change in family relationships resulting in the increase of family system resources (e.g. flexibility of control, an increase in the adaptation skills of the family for changing reality, an increase in security through adequate role fulfillment, the reinforcement of clear communication, an increase in the adequacy of expressed feelings, building emotional bonds, and growth of tolerance for various systems of values within family members)[2] ; 3) change of self-activity perception (acceptance of personal responsibility for all acts connected with violence and creation of a plan of action to prevent violence in future); 4) making oneself aware of the impact of violence on one's life through discovery of one's own bits and pieces of experience from childhood.

The therapy I proposed consisted of several phases. The first phase was to make participants aware of the harm which they did to their intimates. To achieve this, there were a number of tasks to be performed such as defining the violence (which types of conduct and their consequences should be qualified as violence) and analyzing one's behavior in the active phase of the disease and after starting the treatment. The second phase involved identifying denial mechanisms and identifying types of conduct aimed at denial. Tasks on which participants worked individually aimed at creating a personal list of kinds of conduct used for denying the application of violence and harming others. The list was supposed to aid recognition of present violence and behaviors related to avoiding responsibility for their violent actions. In this phase of psychotherapy, addicted people concentrate on identifying the feeling of guilt and shame connected with their conduct, beliefs and thoughts concerning these feelings. It was the beginning of realizing personal strategies of action used in difficult situations and recognizing situations which could affect alcohol disease recurrence[3]. The next phase of psychotherapy aimed at deepening the awareness of personal experience connected with experiencing violence during one's lifetime, with special emphasis on the childhood phase. The participants analyzed their family relations, relations with peers and other people in their lives in connection with experiencing violence. This stage was associated with the discovery of true feelings and emotions (fear, helplessness, and worries) and searching for their influence on later life. Work on the history of one's life allowed participants to integrate the vision of themselves as both perpetrators and victims of violence. This also let them develop empathy through discovering feelings of shame, harm and hopelessness (Mellibruda, 1995). The next phase of psychotherapy referred to the preparation of compensation for the damage done to intimates. The aim of this phase was to prepare the subject to ask the family to write a letter "In what way did you hurt me" and to accept "the truth" about experiencing pain inflicted by an alcoholic. The aim of the last, fifth phase was to prepare a plan of making up for the damage and confirming it with people that were hurt.

The psychotherapy planned in this manner was accomplished in seven therapeutic groups from 2002 to 2009. Seventy-three persons took part.

Therapy conduct

It can be said that participants were well motivated to take part in therapy because of a strong stimulus to improve their relationships with people they cared about. Taking part in the therapy and experiencing its positive effects in every day life, especially in relations with people, had an important influence on motivation. People who decided to continue the process of getting sober especially in the aspect of violence could anticipate positive changes deriving from their actions. In some cases motivation was based on external factors and associated with fear of divorce. On the basis of conversations with participants it can be suggested that their anticipations connected with the aims of therapy concurred with the aims planned by the therapist. In spite of their fear to confront themselves with their violent activity, they decided to enter into a therapeutic deal.

During the psychotherapy the patients revealed their violent behaviors openly and willingly; they identified and recognized negation at the cognitive level. They often verbally expressed their willingness to work on violent behaviors concerning not only family members but also other people and animals. However, the difficulty was in confronting their own responsibility connected with the feeling of guilt. Numerous addicted persons still tried to justify their actions and denied the fact that they were guilty. Most often, such justifications were used as: *it's not me, it's the alcohol* and *she wasn't without guilt as well.* Often such statements occurred: *I am OK now, I stopped drinking and this is what bothered them (family) most* or another statement *why do we have to rub salt into the wound? it is well now.* Working with the aid of violent conduct forced the addicted persons to omit some forms of violence, e.g. sexual violence. Omission took the form of forgetting, which led to no admission of the task. Such behavior occurred to many people when the task referred to sexual violence. Participants said that they did not remember any conduct which would lead to sexual violence. At meetings when one of the participants took the risk of disclosing this area of behavior, other people also started disclosing their own similar activities. In the course of presenting individual admissions, some people minimized the effects of their behavior, or did not disclose factual situations. Mechanisms of under-estimation, minimization or irony were applied particularly heavily among numerous forms of disclosing defensive mechanisms. One example was the joke about performed violence. One participant said:

> *of course I was unfaithful to my wife but she should have been satisfied as I was off her head. I did not come back home for nights, she didn't have to watch me drunk.*

Another person said:

> *when I was drinking, I did not hurt anybody, basically I do not know why I enrolled in this program, probably out of curiosity. My family did not suffer any harm due to my drinking. When I came back tipsy, I was very entertaining. I joked with my wife and children. Especially my son liked to play with me, we fooled around together with ease and there was a lot of fun. When I was more than drunk, I went to bed and my wife stayed with the children and watched television. (...) We were close to each other, as when my son fell off the stairs and made his head bleed, we went together to the hospital.*

The above-provided statements refer to the first stage of therapy. The same participants in the course of subsequent meetings discovered significant facts proving their use of violence towards their relatives and closest family. Working through the history of one's life and discovering one's own experiences related to being a victim of violence was an important stage of the therapy. The participants gained further insight into the mechanisms of violence and feelings experienced by victims.

The second critical moment referred to the stage when patients received letters describing experienced pain or injury from their families. Many people were more than surprised by these stories and tried to defend themselves with statements like: "*she wasn't without guilt as well*" or "*it was not quite so*". At this moment it is worth providing some fragments of letters written by close people as they confirmed various forms of behavior as victims and their active or passive conduct. One of the wives wrote:

> *What you have done was awful. I never knew what would happen. When you did not come back home at 5pm, it was clear to me that you will come back late in the evening and interrogation will start. It went on for hours. I remember that at one time I was ill but you drunk-dragged me out of bed and ordered me to sit on a stool in the middle of our kitchen. I was sitting for several hours and shivered with cold while you were shouting at me that I am hopeless and cannot run the house and make you happy. Then you were only mumbling. When I tried to stand up, you were pushing me so that I sat down again and you shouted some more so that I could not listen to you. You stopped only in the morning.*

Another person wrote:

> *When you were drunk, you behaved awful. You were calling me names and often you said our older daughter was the same kind of who... as her mum. You checked her exercise books at 4.00 in the morning tore her books to pieces and scattered them all over the room. We both were terrified. You did not even let our dog sleep. You threw him out on frosty nights or kicked him. At one time I together with Ann had to run away from home, as you came back and started shattering furniture. I was afraid you would kill us all.*

Another person described the passive character of violence very expressively:

> *It is true that while you were drinking there were never any quarrels but there was no contact with you as well. When I was ill, you were not with me. Of course you were, but drunk lying in the other room. It was our daughter who was 8 then who ran to our neighbours and called the ambulance. You did not visit me at the hospital as well, as you were afraid of meeting my mother. Once when drunk, you insisted on hanging drapes, you climbed onto a stool and fell down. I was petrified as blood was running out of your head and you lost consciousness. Another time you fell down the stairs and broke your nose. I had to continuously take care of you.*

But still family members described the present situation in such a way that gives evidence of repeated occurrences of various kinds of violence:

> *since you started treatment nothing has changed, maybe just that you do not drink. I am still afraid of you. I do know how you will react to my worse school grade or if I ask for money. I can see that you changed you behavior but your bad moods, explosions of anger or not speaking to us mean that I cannot feel safe. A month ago you made a row that we spent too much money and called us spongers and that we spent your money so*

> *easily, without taking anything into consideration. I can never count on you. Some days ago I wanted you to drive me to my friend's as I was feeling bad, then you were mad and wriggled out of it saying that you have got other tasks to do. Then all evening you were gabbing that I make use of you and that my mother was right that she went away.*

Another person wrote:

> *I am glad that I can write it all to you. (...) Now when you do not drink, it is not any better. Happily I go to Al-anon sessions, as otherwise I could not bear it. (...) You expect sex from me but think that it is my duty. You are not interested if I am ready for it. I feel sick when you tell me to "have a shower" as I know what it means that I have to fulfill your sexual fantasies. After everything you turn your back and fall asleep and then I feel disgust. We never talk about it as for you it is not a problem. It is similar with other issues. It is to be so as you wish it; I am not taken into consideration. You behave like a lout. All you can do is criticise me and never say anything good. You reproach me when I do something. I invited my cousin last Saturday, and then you got furious that you cannot rest at home as all the time somebody is there and disturbs you. We were sitting in the other room, so as not to disturb you and I was shivering with anxiety if you would make a row in her presence or not. Then you turned the TV up so that we could not talk and sprawled all over our couch with a newspaper. I felt ashamed.*

An example of planned activities connected with atonement was that:

1. all the participants were working on preparations to ask their families to forgive them for any harm they had done to them;
2. any participant having any problems with anger was to take part in the therapy for people with this problem;
3. another person planned to ask his family for forgiveness and was preparing to have a talk on current problems;
4. a person who had problems with keeping in contact with his children planned to work on gaining skills to support his daughters in various life situations and increase his empathy;
5. a person who had avoided responsibility for the family situation with his harmful escapades was to take part in a therapeutic program for victims of domestic violence;
6. a person who manifested humiliating behavior toward close family friends was to build respect towards other people by helping with housework.

Implementation of the programs created by participants covered two stages. The first one covered three months starting from the end of the therapy and included tasks focused mainly on building relations with relatives and closest family friends through co-operation in taking on real-life tasks. The second stage covered a half year in getting sober and referred to gaining new skills by compensating for having shown pain and suffering, e.g. displaying empathy, showing emotions, coping with anger, and listening to others.

Evaluation of the process of change

Contact with the partner of an addicted person and getting her to co-operate was a significant element of the therapy offered. Co-operation was based on taking part in an interview that analyseds the violence (a list of violent kinds of conduct) [4] before the beginning of the psychotherapy and after it had ended. During the interview, the therapist encouraged family members to start their own therapy as victims of domestic abuse.

Before starting the psychotherapy, disclosure of convictions on doubts and fears relating to violence in family relations was an important element of the interview. On one hand, they claimed that being hurt by the alcoholic during the active phase of the disease and during its treatment is a significant problem that made every-day contact difficult; on the other hand, they expressed unwillingness to touch upon this topic during their conversations with an alcoholic. They stated that such a conversation and confrontation would not change anything and that it might provoke the alcoholic to go back to drinking and continue family conflicts. Simultaneously the very same persons admitted that during domestic conflicts and disagreements they often shouted out, sometimes in a very vulgar manner, all the alcoholic's wrongdoings to show him what an awful tyrant and abuser he was and is. After the end of the therapy for domestic-violence perpetrators, the problem of "the past" became less overwhelming. Partners of alcoholics indicated that it was easier for them to understand mechanisms of negation and the hiding of experiences relating to violence both by themselves and an alcoholic. The very fact that an alcoholic was working on his / her violent activity was a factor which minimized willingness to make excuses and therefore to further burden an alcoholic with responsibility for having done harm to others. Partners noticed that alcoholics are aware of both their guilt and responsibility for the recovery of family relations. Changes evaluated with the aid of the interview with family members demonstrated that physical violence had been eliminated thoroughly, and verbal and economical violence - to a considerable degree.

Research on the psychotherapy of alcoholics as perpetrators of domestic violence

There is little research on the effectiveness of psychotherapy on alcoholics as domestic violence perpetrators, because the topic is not a separate branch of psychology. Some advice on treating it specifically is given by the authors analyzing BCT (Behavioral Couples Therapy), who indicate the significant role of working on marital relationships in an alcoholic's family and the positive effects of this work (O'Farrell, 1999; O'Farrell, Murphy, 1995; O'Farrell, Van Hutton, Murphy, 1999).

The proposition of my therapy supplements alcohol addiction therapy and shows the complexity of the problem of violence in alcoholic families during both the active phase of illness and its treatment (Dyjakon, 2006). The difficulties with the evaluation of therapy effectiveness are connected with the influence of numerous beyond-therapeutic factors on the life of therapy participants. While analyzing differences, only families without significant changes (serious illness, loss of work, partners splitting up, and promotion at work) should have been considered in order to avoid behavior and relations falsification.

Conclusions

Therapy indicates that addicted people in confronting their violence find it to be a very difficult task even if they were previous participants of alcohol addiction therapy. At the same time, changes which are effected by the therapy seem to lead to a growing sense of "normality" in alcoholic families and also seem to lower the tension resulting from unsolved problems. The knowledge and skills gained by participants during therapy started to be new family resources which allow them to solve difficult situations in an assertive manner.

Notes

[1] http://www.policja.pl/portal/pol/4/318/Przemoc_w_rodzinie.html (verified 2010-01-03 12:01:43)

[2] following W. Świętochowski "Systemowa analiza wybranych uwarunkowań radzenia sobie ze stresem" in: "Zeszyty Naukowe WSHE w Łodzi nr 2 (15)/2001"

[3] Following Woronicz, the recurrence of alcohol disease is comprehended as coming back to thinking, feeling and acting similar to the active stage of the disease.

[4] The list of violent forms of conduct was prepared by the author of the research.

CHAPTER FOURTEEN

TRAUMA IN THE WORK OF A SEXOLOGIST: SELF-EXPERIENCED AND THAT EXPERIENCED BY OTHERS

MARIA BEISERT

Introduction

The work of a sexologist, similar to the work of any other person in a profession of social trust, results in specific, though not exclusively positive or negative, outcomes.

What is so special about this profession that would allow one to expect consequences that are different from other professions of social trust? There are three aspects worth noting. The first, less explored aspect, is related to the consequences of frequent (continuous) exposure to sexual stimuli. The distinctive feature is the content of the communication between the sexologist with the patient, namely the sexual content that first becomes the subject of diagnosis and then of therapy. Studies of the consequences of continuous exposure to sexual material are scarce. Some of them focus on the negative and distant consequences of this exposure in the form of unethical behavior on the part of the sexologist toward the patient (Lew-Starowicz, 2000). Other studies concentrate on the effects directly related to the intimate functioning of the sexologist, in the form of altered perception of sexual stimuli, changes in beliefs or reactivity (Figley, 1995). They include the therapist's withdrawal from close relationships (sexual relationships), caused by the therapist's perception that no one is able to be a partner of a person who deals with the dark side of the human sexuality. The sense of one's own uniqueness in turn intensifies the impression of distance and deprives the person of his or her chance for a happy relationship with people who encounter a wide range of sexual reactions, not only with the disturbed. The end result is described in literature (Dutton and Rubinstein, 1995): seclusion in one's own professional circle, among the only people whose experiences are similar, and distancing oneself from diversity and closeness of others.

The second type of consequence results from the place sexuality is ascribed in the hierarchy of values of individuals and societies. It is a taboo sphere, regarded as a strictly personal, intimate area. The problems hidden in this sphere may therefore differ to a significant degree-due to their drastic and bizarre nature-from emotional or social problems. Sexual disturbances for many patients pose a threat to self-esteem and to their body image, as well as risking social isolation, loss of social esteem or even of freedom. This fact results in more rigid and complex defense mechanisms employed by individuals. Thus both the form and the content make the work with patients difficult for the sexologist. Coming into contact with them by definition means coming into contact with their negative emotions, high emotional tension, and, which usually means, working in stressful conditions. Even more difficult may be to work therapeutically with persons who constantly experience the results of their past sexual traumas (drastic forms of sexual abuse, sexual contacts with persons whose sexual preferences were disturbed, rapes or tortures) (Beisert, 2008). Touching upon the untreated trauma entails pain and suffering. It brings about certain well known and inevitable-that does not mean destructive-consequences for the therapists. These phenomena apply more working with victims than they do to working with abusers, although, as we will see further on, that is not entirely obvious. Finally, the third difference that places the work of a sexologist at a high level of difficulty boils down to the fact that sexuality is the subject of many norms (legal, moral, religious) that do not necessarily constitute a consistent, common system (for both parties of the diad patient-therapist). The necessity of respecting the norms, and, moreover, taking into consideration specific barriers resulting from religious beliefs or social conventions, makes it difficult to offer help that complies to the standards and capabilities available within the framework of contemporary sex therapeutic knowledge. These reasons simultaneously not only determine the occurrence of certain risk factors related to working in this profession but also determine specific protective factors.

Factors that increase the risk of negative consequences of working as a sexologist

Exposure to another person's trauma

Many authors have directly posed the question whether continuous contact with material related to sexual abuse and sexual cruelty exposes the therapist to the risk of negative phenomena related to their work.

Research by Kadambi et al. (2004) proved that not only is the risk no higher than it is in the case of work with oncology patients, but also that it is not higher than the risk involved in general psychological practice. The authors' interpretation aims at showing that there is likely a peculiar pre-selection of persons, who undertake therapeutic work with victims of trauma, or else that therapists use efficient ways of coping with the requirements they are confronted with, and therefore most professionals (including sexual therapists) do not experience, for example, trauma by proxy. These objective results, however, were not in accordance with the results describing the impressions of therapists. Therapists who encounter sexual violence on a daily basis assessed their field as decisively exposing them to secondary traumatisation. Such assessment was given by 83% of sex therapists examined, while 50% of psychologists working with people suffering from cancer, and 36% of general psychologists reported this risk. Thus, according to subjective data, exposure to another person's trauma of sexual nature is a risk factor on its own.

An entirely different view, in accordance with therapists' subjective experiences, is manifested by a significant group of researchers, documenting it through empirical data. Results prove that working with patients who expose their therapists to sexual trauma (irrespective of whether the patient was the abuser or the abused) constitutes a serious risk of negative psychological consequences. Farrenkopf (1992) in his study described the mental health of therapists working with sexual offenders. Approximately one-third of the subjects manifested high levels of vigilance, suspiciousness and excessive concern for their security, and treated these symptoms as consequences of their practice. Moreover, twenty percent of the subjects reported high levels of generalised stress, exhaustion, depression and professional burn-out.

On the other hand, Schauben and Frazier (1995) noted a risk (besides PTSD symptoms) to the cognitive patterns of the therapists working with other people's (sexual) traumas. The alterations in cognitive patterns pertained to the therapists themselves and to other people. The symptoms of secondary trauma in female therapists working with large numbers of clients who had experienced sexual trauma in their past were described by Brady, Guy, Poelstra and Brokaw (1995).

Pearlman and Mac Ian (1995) examined 188 therapists working with traumatized patients and found high levels of stress, intrusive thoughts and avoidance, and a disturbed perception of security and trust. Confirmation of these results was provided by a study by Kassan-Adams (1995), showing that one hundred therapists working with patients who were sexual trauma victims manifested symptoms of avoidance and intrusions that significantly correlated with exposure to their patients' traumas. This way of describing the threats resulting from work with another person's trauma is supported in the studies on symptoms occurring in therapists working with victims of torture (Lansen, 2001). Contact with PTSD symptoms triggered such behaviors as systematic extension of stress onto the whole team and mobbing towards co-workers.

Very interesting results come from other studies concerning the problem of exposure to trauma that treat it as a factor with a more complex impact. These are studies of therapists working with persons who experienced trauma and who in the process of intervention employed a method called "working through trauma" (Deighton, Gurris and Traue, 2007). This type of intervention involved continuous exposure to extremely dramatic stimulus situations (including torture) that were part of the patient's experience. On the one hand, the study was designed to estimate whether such extensive exposure is associated with professional burn-out, compassion fatigue and secondary trauma while, on the other hand, the authors were seeking to establish links between specific conditions of the exposure, variables pertaining to the subjects of the study (approval of the methods of working through trauma, that is, the extent to which it is employed) and the negative, above-mentioned results. In the course of the first stage of research it was found that compassion fatigue, symptoms of professional burn-out, and high levels of stress co-occurred with low rates of working though trauma. Therapists with low rates of working through trauma (and thus less likely to be at risk of exposure to drastic stimuli) suffered more negative consequences than those who were exposed to such contact regularly. The result did not confirm the existence of a direct positive correlation of exposure to trauma with negative consequences perceived by the therapists, all the more so because there was a significant discrepancy between therapists recognizing the discussed method of working through trauma as the required one and the matter of actually employing it.

An approach to working with trauma victims

The results gathered by a team of three researchers, Deighton, Gurris, and Traue (2007), were elaborated and repeated during another stage of the research. This time it was not only the exposure to other persons' traumas that was the focus of the study, but the conformity between the actual employment of the method of working through trauma (namely the actual contact with the patient's trauma) and approval of it. The subjects were divided into three groups: S (Success - high level of approval of the method of working through trauma and high level of employment of the method), F (Frustration - high level of approval and low level of employment of the method), and N (Non-Advocacy - low level of method advocacy and low level of employment of the method). It was at this point that the authors discovered that trauma by proxy, compassion fatigue, PTSD symptoms and somatisation, and moreover, professional burn-out in an indirect way, occurred exclusively among therapists belonging to the F group. This group of therapists openly advocated the method of working through trauma, but reported such high rates of obstacles in employing it that they very infrequently dealt with trauma. This data shows that what matters is not so much the exposure to trauma as the way the therapist acts when confronted with the content of it. The subjects from group F were in contact with patients, witnessed their activities, knew their history and the course of their trauma, and advocated the necessity of working through it. However, they themselves evaded actions. Their anxiety manifesting itself in avoidance was recognized as a factor reinforcing the symptoms of anxiety in patients and therapists alike, leading to a peculiar cooperation in avoidance. For therapists, the avoidance accompanied by acceptance of the necessity to utilize the chosen method meant discrepancy between beliefs and behaviors, and lack of any possibility to adapt their behavior to demands put upon them. The discomfort caused by this situation was the source of secondary trauma, compassion fatigue, burn-out and additional symptoms. None of these experiences occurred in those cases where the subjects belonged to the remaining two groups. The S group were exposed to trauma during their work, but were not at risk of avoidance and discrepancy. The development of adverse symptoms was prevented by active confrontation with trauma together with the patient, and by the satisfaction of showing him or her compassion. This conclusion was confirmed by the results pertaining to the N group, where decisively abstaining from the unaccepted method and not exposing oneself to its ambivalence reduced the risk of the discussed negative results.

Even though they did not pertain exclusively to sexual trauma (only some forms of torture were of this nature), the quoted studies allowed for the understanding of the significance of exposure to trauma in the work of a sex therapist. What was revealed as the most important factor was not the exposure to trauma itself but the ability and internal motivation of the therapist to confront its content. The key role was played by the discrepancy between beliefs and behavior of the therapist along with the underlying anxiety of being exposed to trauma, or rather of actively working it through.

Conclusions from other studies inform us that these results are not accidental. Linley and Joseph (2007) proved that a professional background, specifically the type of paradigm within the framework of which the therapists were conducting their work with trauma victims, is of great significance with respect to the results of their work. The comparison of cognitive-behavioral therapists with humanistic or transpersonal therapists showed that the former find less positive elements in their work and register lower rates of personal development, showing more symptoms of professional burn-out. The authors of the study believe that the other two groups of therapists base their work on theories that promote such values as personal growth, overcoming one's limitations, significance of the sense of community, and cooperation in achieving success. These theories facilitate attaining these aims for therapists and sustain them in their striving to help the persons in need. Moreover, it is likely that the behavioral therapist's situation is made more difficult by such factors as matching specific groups of patients (offenders and the intellectually handicapped), matching specific groups of symptoms (violence, manipulation, severe and chronic symptoms), and matching specific expectations (short contracts and results measurable by means of external indicators to the paradigm). In this case it would mean that the paradigms allowing for deeper therapeutic work protect against exposure to trauma, which explicitly confirms the conclusions arising from the formerly cited studies.

Similar conclusions arise from studies on professional burn-out and secondary trauma occurring in specialists diagnosing sexually abused children (Perron and Hiltz, 2006). Persons who interview children for the courts (collecting information about their abuse) did not manifest any symptoms of sexual abuse or trauma, even though their work consisted exclusively of exposure to other person's sexual trauma. It was also found that their personal characteristics did not correlate with the discussed phenomena. Explanation of these results was sought in the nature of the relationship between the victim and the interviewer. The process of information acquisition was at least partially structuralized, limited in time, and objectified, which significantly reduced intimacy, preventing the occurrence of any emotional relationship between the participants involved. In turn, the absence of a bond prevented the professional from getting involved in the child's problem. As to how intense the impact of a deep bond with the trauma victim can be (causing an increase in satisfaction derived from showing compassion), we are informed about by the studies on the positive influence of this variable on the wellbeing of the therapist (Linley and Joseph, 2007).

The cited studies show that exposure to another person's trauma itself does not determine its effect on the professional and personal life of a sex therapist. It is only the motivation to work with the content of the trauma and the therapist's mode of working with it (the depth and the bond) that constitute good prognostic factors bringing hope for success.

Trauma in a sexologist's life history

The results of a sex therapist's work are also determined - apart from the specificity of the field - by specific subjective and situational factors. As there are numerous studies extensively documenting the influence of the above-mentioned factors on the life and work of therapists, I shall at this point focus my attention on a lesser known element, namely trauma in the life history of the therapist who works with other people's traumas.

The therapist's own trauma (particularly sexual trauma) is sometimes regarded an obstacle in working with a patient, as it generates the risk of "exploiting" him or her for the purpose of coping with the therapist's personal trauma. Simultaneously, the presence of the therapist's own painful experience may intensify the symptoms of burn-out, secondary trauma and compassion fatigue. This line of reasoning was empirically confirmed. Pearlman and Mac Ian (1995) studied 188 therapists and found that those who had experienced trauma in their history and later worked with traumatised patients manifested higher levels of stress, intrusive thoughts and avoidance, as well as a disturbed perception of danger and trust. Similarly, research conducted by Kassan-Adams (1995) proved that one hundred therapists working with patients who experienced sexual trauma manifested symptoms of avoidance and intrusion that significantly correlated with exposure to their patients' trauma. The therapists' own trauma, as in case of the above-discussed study, was found to be an important predictor of PTSD-like symptoms manifested by the therapists. In the study by Kadambi et al. (2004) it was found that a significant rate of therapists (58.2%) experienced trauma (as it is defined in DSM-IV) in their history, and this correlated negatively with the results in the scales measuring trauma by proxy. There is also other, more recent data (Deighton, Gurris and Traue, 2007) demonstrating that the impact of the presence of a trauma in the therapists' history (all therapists in the study worked with trauma victims) was unidirectional, causing such symptoms as secondary traumatic stress, compassion fatigue, professional burn-out, disturbance of cognitive patterns, intrusions, and a high level of distress. In all the cited studies, the therapist's own trauma was regarded as a permanent handicap that restricted, though did not exclude, the ability to work. Such a resolute and deterministic way of understanding the role of trauma in life would only accept a destructive or impairing influence of trauma, totally excluding from the discussion the developmental significance of hardships and suffering for the further functioning of a human being. The concept of secondary trauma stress suggests that the personal history of a therapist may be a high risk factor in those cases where the therapist's exposure to another person's trauma is long term.

On the other hand, a study conducted almost simultaneously (Schauben and Frazier, 1995) by means of regression analysis shows that counselors (148 women) victimized in their history did not show any higher rates of stress as a result of work with survivors (of sexual trauma) than the counselors without a history of trauma. Similar results acquired from a different population (156 therapists, some of whom did not work with trauma victims), reveal a similar phenomenon. Here we learn that the personal experience of trauma did not increase the risk of secondary dramatization, and, moreover, it did contribute to personal growth. Simultaneously, what was found to be predictive of personal growth and positive change perceived by the therapists was the participation (current and previous) in one's own therapy and formal supervision. However, a comparison of reports by therapists who had experienced trauma, and those who were not traumatized and never underwent any therapy, showed significant differences between them, to the advantage of reports of trauma survivors (a higher rate of participation). Subjects who underwent therapy were characterized by lower rates of professional burn-out, experienced positive changes resulting form their work, and regarded their personal growth as significantly better. These recent results pointing to the role of therapy in the work with trauma victims explain the meaning of trauma in the therapists' lives in a different way than the former group of studies did. Here the therapist's own trauma may be a developmental advantage. Collins and Long (2003), in explaining this phenomenon, refer to the possibility of using one's own personal experience. According to them, due to this experience the therapists' feelings arising in response to contact with another person's trauma may be treated more maturely. These therapists more frequently apply positive coping strategies which they learned while working through their own trauma.

However, the comparison of different results arising from these two studies does not lead to any definite conclusions. First, a comment is required on the selection of subjects for the studied groups. In the studies where the results definitely point to a person's own history as a risk factor, the groups constituted mostly (but not exclusively) of therapists who worked with trauma victims. However, extensive and well documented research conducted by Linley and Joseph (2007) examined the wellbeing of a large group of therapists, but (who) were not required to work with trauma victims. This factor, as well as undergoing their own psychotherapy, allows one to differently interpret the influence on therapists of working with trauma victims. It is likely indeed that being a trauma victim increases the risk of compassion fatigue or the risk of symptoms of stress by proxy in situations of continuous exposure to stimuli similar to the ones experienced in the past. This would be confirmed by the results focusing on one type of therapist and one aspect of their job. However, the final influence of the history of one's life is modified by mediatory variables: the way a person copes with his or her own trauma - which can be tentatively concluded from the content of the above paragraph -, the type of paradigm employed in therapeutic work, the motivation to undertake the work, and the bond with the patient. The negative life experience of a therapist may be useful for both the sake of personal growth of the therapist and his or her patient.

Factors protecting the sexologists' health and wellbeing

An interesting perspective for sexual therapists is revealed by research on positive phenomena relating to the work with sexual pathologies, that is, research on compassion satisfaction and self-care. Both factors are regarded as preventing burn-out and fatigue (Stamm, 1998; Kraus, 2005).

The notion of satisfaction stemming from compassion was discussed for the first time in the analysis and research by Stamm (1998), although the question as to what the therapists gain from working with trauma victims, with the drastic material constituting the residue of their past experience, or continuous exposure to sexual pathologies, had already been posed to therapists in the past. Research by Schauben and Frazier (1995) led to isolating the following factors: participation in the process of change and recovery, observation of strength, and creativity and resilience in others, particularly in persons as seriously harmed as the victims of sexual abuse are. These elements (discussed most frequently) referred to traits or processes allocated in the patients, while being the source of positive experiences for the therapists. Less frequently mentioned were the therapists' traits and states in this role, for example a sense of the importance of their work. Stamm (ibidem), who noticed that some therapists who intensively employ compassion in their work do not react with fatigue to the need of continuously showing it to their patients, has clearly defined the notion of compassion. Compassion consists in feeling and acting with deep empathy and sadness towards the suffering of other people, and it is necessary, though not sufficient in itself, in the work of a therapist. What the author regarded as important and necessary is not acting with empathy itself, but the motivation to act this way, that is, to draw satisfaction from participating in the process of helping others. The two-component definition of compassion (the feeling component plus the motivation to act on it) allows one to better understand why for some people helping others is tiring, while for others it is something that enables them to function with prolonged satisfaction. The helpers want to help - among other reasons - because it gives them satisfaction (in literature called compassion satisfaction). This prevents them from resigning from their work, despite the risk of suffering exposure to stress and abuse.

The recent work of Stamm (2002) confirmed this prediction. The satisfaction felt by persons working with trauma victims correlated negatively with professional burn-out and compassion fatigue. The subjects reported that the main sources of this satisfaction were being part of a team pursuing a common idea in a spirit of comradeship and cooperation, accompanying others in their growth and recovery, giving support, and supervising the recovery.

Self-care, variously conceptualised and operationalized, is also treated as an important element that reduces the negative influence of the work performed. The best example is research done on the coping processes which proved that active strategies of coping with stress used by counselors and therapists reduce the risk of negative effects of helping. Seeking various forms of support and planning and using humor correlated negatively with the occurrence of the PTSD-like symptoms of compassion fatigue, experiencing negative affects and burn-out. Similar outcomes were brought about by other particular strategies, such as adequate sleep, nutrition, meditation, reading, having a circle of reliable friends, the possibility of getting advice, and support from close others. The studies and analysis by Stamm (1998, 2002) allow one to view, with some optimism, the work of sexologists who work with sometimes extremely severe forms of sexual abuse.

Similar questions, though viewing the difficulties of working in the field of human sexuality from a different perspective, are answered by studies on therapists working with sexual offenders. Kraus (2005) examined ninety clinicians working with juvenile sexual offenders, and for this reason participated in various therapeutic programs conducted in Oregon. The major research objective was to establish the answer to the question of whether self-care manifested by clinicians (therapists) contributes to the reduction of compassion fatigue and professional burn-out, and increases satisfaction experienced as a result of compassion showed to other people. The measurement of variables by means of questionnaire methods led to an interesting result, illustrated in Table 5-1.

Table 14-1 Coefficient Alphas and Correlations between Scales

Type of variable	alpfa	1.	2.	3.
1. Self care	.88			
2. Burnout	.80	.16		
3. Compassion satisfaction	.87	.46*	-.43*	
4. Compassion fatigue	.85	.12	.65*	-.20
N=90 *p<.01 Source: Kraus, 2005				

Three of the regularities found in the Table are worth noting. First, it is revealed in the Table that a therapist's self-care and the satisfaction derived from compassion shown to patients are correlated positively. It does not mean, however, that one may say anything about the order of cause and effect. Individuals that take care of themselves, meaning that they use effective strategies for coping with stress (not necessarily professional stress), for utilizing support, turning to friends for advice, and to supervisors for feedback are also those who do not accumulate stress, apply themselves to their work with energy, and are able to enjoy their achievements, including the fact that while fulfilling their obligations, they are giving support to others and offering them compassion. Obviously, it is not difficult to imagine an opposite situation where the satisfaction drawn from the work is the motivation-to give oneself care and attention that is to self-care.

Second, research has shown that professional burn-out correlates positively with compassion fatigue and negatively with satisfaction. It may be that it is satisfaction that protects against burn-out and increases self-care. It is curious that compassion fatigue and compassion satisfaction were not dependent on one another in any significant way. The observed dependency points to a certain tendency, but the result does not entitle us to a statement that satisfaction counterbalances the compassion fatigue.

Third, it was found that, unfortunately, self-care does not reduce in any significant way professional burn-out and compassion fatigue, as if self-care itself was an insufficient buffer against them. It may be that the relationship of self-care with satisfaction points to an indirect influence of self-care, or to the greater significance of satisfaction for counteracting negative phenomena in the work process. Care in reference to the therapist (his or her well-being, interpersonal contacts, and relieving tension or solving problems) may not include such an important element of preventing negative phenomena related to work as information from a human being (the patient). It is only the observation of his or her states, the processes of recovery or of the general positive change that constitutes the decisive element for the assessment of the outcomes of the work. The significance of this element, which is the significance of information coming from the other participants of therapy, is probably an important element that averts the risk of burn-out and fatigue. One may hypothesize that the first protective factor, namely self-care, constitutes the basis for satisfaction (which is confirmed by the correlation between them: .46). This result also points to the necessity of seeking a key to preventing the negative effects of working as a therapist in the equilibrium or in the integrated impact of two classes of factors: those directly related to the therapist (self-care), and those that are related to the patient (possibility to participate in positive changes). The essence of the sex therapist's profession is to help in recovery, in discarding pathologies, facilitating growth and reaching wellbeing. Without recognizing the importance of this activity, it is hard to imagine that the therapy would be successful and efficient. It is the participation in the processes involved in therapy, not only the end result that is responsible for perceived satisfaction. Thus the therapist's concern about him- or herself and their wellbeing on its own does not prevent negative outcomes of their profession. On the other hand, focusing on the second of the buffers (satisfaction from showing compassion to other people) is not sufficient. What testifies to this is the weak correlation between satisfaction and compassion fatigue, as well as the results of other studies, indicative of the danger of viewing a therapist's state (that is, the absence of burn-out) as depending exclusively on the outcomes of his or her work with the patient (even when measured solely by participation in the process).

Conclusion

Certainly, the above analysis of a few selected aspects of the sexologist's work constitutes inadequate material for any generalizations. However, the collected pieces of data (at times totally contradictory) have revealed a certain picture. Sexologists come into contact with the domains of taboo and pathology, both verging on criminal offence. And this is the part of their work that determines the gravity of the profession. To cut the discussion short, one may say that there are two important conclusions among the ones discussed above. It is the subjective impression of the weight of the responsibilities (unquestionably shown by Kadambi (2007), and the significance of compassion satisfaction for the profession. It shows to what extent the subjective senses of burden and fatigue are able to waste the work and effort in every profession. On the other hand, the feeling of satisfaction convinces that the motivation to change the world in the direction of "improvement" may be helpful in bearing the hardest professional experiences, even those that undermine our faith in ideals and in human nature, no matter how they are described.

BIBLIOGRAPHY

Agrawal, H., Gunderson, J., Holmes, B., Lyons-Ruth, K. 2004. Attachment studies with borderline patients: a review. Harvard Review of Psychiatry, 12, 94-104.

Allard, C. 2009. Prevalence and sequelae of betrayal trauma in Japanese student Sample. Psychological Trauma: Theory, Research, Practice, and Policy, Vol. S (1), 65-177.

Allen, J. 2001. Traumatic relationships and serious mental disorders. New York: Wiley & Sons, Ltd.

Allen, B., Lauterbach, D. 2007. Personality characteristics of adult survivors of childhood trauma. Journal of Traumatic Stress, 20 (4): 587-595.

American Psychiatric Association. 1980. Diagnostic and statistical manual of mental disorders. (3rd ed.). Washington, DC: American Psychiatric Association.

American Psychiatric Association. 1994. Diagnostic and statistical manual of mental disorders. (4th ed.). Revised. Washington, DC: American Psychiatric Association.

—. 2000. Diagnostic and statistical manual of mental disorders. (4rt ed. TR). Washington, DC: American Psychiatric Association.

Andersson, B., Nilsson, S. 1964. Studies in the reliability and validity of the critical incident technique. Journal of Applied Psychology, 48, 398-403.

Andrews, B. 1995. Bodily shame as a mediator between abusive experiences and depression. Journal of Abnormal Psychology, 104: 277-285.

Argenti, N., Schramm, K. 2009. Remembering Violence: Antropological Perspectives on Intergenerational Transmission. Berghahn Books.

Aronson, E., Wilson, T., Akert, R. 1997. Psychologia społeczna. Serce i umysł. [Social Psychology. Heart and Mind.]. Poznań: Wydawnictwo Zysk i S-ka.

Badura – Madej, W., Dobrzyńska – Mesterhazy, A. 2000. Przemoc w rodzinie. Interwencja kryzysowa i psychoterapia. [Violence in the family. Crisis intervention and psychotherapy.]. Kraków: Wydawnictwo Uniwersytetu Jagiellońskiego.

Badura-Madej, W., Dobrzyńska-Mesterhazy, A. 2000. Przemoc w rodzinie.

Interwencja kryzysowa i psychoterapia. [Violence in the family. Crisis intervention and psychotherapy.]. Kraków: Wydawnictwo UJ.

Baker, L. 1984. Treating Couples in Crisis. Fundamentals and Practice in Marital Therapy. London: The Free Press.

Bandura, A. 1973. Aggression: A social learning analysis. Englewood Cliffs: NJ: Prentice-Hall.

Baradell, J., Klein, K. 1993. Relationship of life stress and body consciousness to hypervigilant decision making. Journal of Personality and Social Psychology, 64: 267-273.

Baron, R., Richardson, D. 1994. Human aggression. New York: Plenum Press.

Bateson, G. 1991. A sacred Unity- Further Steps to an Ecology of Mind. Harper Colins Publishers.

Bateson, C., Ahmad, N., Stocks, E. 2008. Korzysci i problemy związane z altruizmem wzbudzonym przez empatię. [The benefits and problems associated with altruism excited by empathy.] In A.G. Miller (Ed.), Dobro i zło z perspektywy psychologii społecznej. [Good and evil from the perspective of social psychology]. (pp. 447-479). Kraków: Wydawnictwo WAM.

Battle, C., Shea, T., Johnson, D. 2004. Childhood maltreatment associated with adult personality disorders: findings from the collaborative longitudinal personality disorders study. Journal of Personality Disorders, 18, 193-211.

Becker-Blease, K., Deater-Deckard, K., Eley. 2004. A genetic analysis of individual differences in dissociative behaviors in childhood and adolescence. Journal of Child Psychology and Psychiatry, 45, 522-532.

Beisert, M. 2004. Kazirodztwo. Rodzice w roli sprawców. [Incest. Parents in the role of perpetrators.]. Warszawa: Wydawnictwo Naukowe Scholar.

—. 2008. Incest. Parents as perpetrators. Warsaw: Scholar Scientific Publishing House.

Berkowitz, L. 1972. Social norms, feelings, and other factors affecting helping and altruism. Advances in Experimental Social Psychology, 6, 63-108.

Bernstein, D. P., Fink, L. 1998. Childhood Trauma Questionnaire: A retrospective self-report manual. San Antonio, TX: The Psychological Corporation.

Bidzan, M. 2007. Nastoletnie matki. Psychologiczne aspekty ciąży, porodu i połogu. [Teen Mothers. Psychological Aspects of Pregnancy, Delivery and Puerperium.]. Kraków: Oficyna Wydawnicza „Impuls".

Bion, W.R. 1996. A theory of thinking. In E. Bott Spillius (Ed.), Melanie

Klein Today. Developments in theory and practice. Mainly theory, t. 1, (pp. 178-186). London: Routledge.
Blackburn, R. 2003. Psychopathy and Contribution of Personality to Violence. In T. Millon, E. Simonsen, M. Birket-Smith, R. D. Davie (Eds.), Psychopathy. Antisocial, Criminal and Violent Behavior (pp. 50-68).2387 New York/London: The Guilford Press.
Blatt, S.J., Auerbach, J.S., Levy, K.N. 1997. Mental representations in personality development psychopathology, and the therapeutic process. Review of General Psychology, 1 (4), 351-374.
Boden, J.M., Fergusson, D.M., Horwood, L.J. 2008. Early motherhood and subsequent life outcomes. Journal of Child Psychology and Psychiatry, 49, 151-160.
Bohus, M., Haaf, B., Simms, T. 2004. Effectiveness of inpatient dialectical behavioral therapy for borderline personality disorder: a controlled trial. Behaviour Research and Therapy, 42, 487-499.
Bonanno, G.A. 2008. Loss, trauma, and human resilience: Have we underestimated the human capacity to thrive after extremely aversive events? Psychological Trauma: Theory, Research, Practice, and Policy, Vol. S(1), 101-113.
Boyer, D., Fineman, D., 1992. Sexual abuse as a factor in adolescent pregnancy and child maltreatment. Family Planning Perspectives, 24: 4 - 13.
Bowlby, J. 1973. Attachment and loss, Volume 2: Separaition. New York: Basic Books.
—.1979. The making and Breaking of Affectional Bond. London: Tavistock.
—.1980. Attachment and Loss, Vol. 3: Loses, Sadness and Depression. New York: Basic Books.
—.1988. A secure base: Parent-child attachment and healthy human development. New York: Basic Books.
Brady, J.L., Guy, J.D., Poelstra, P.L., Brokaw, B.F. 1999. Vicarious traumatization, spirituality, and the treatment of sexual abuse survivors: A national survey of women psychotherapists. Professional Psychology: Research and Practice, 30 (4): 386-393.
Bremner, J.D., Innis, R.B., Southwick, S.M., Staib, L., Zoghbi, S. and Charney, D.S. 2000. Decreased benzodiazepine receptor binding in prefrontal cortex in combat-related posttraumatic stress disorder, American Journal of Psychiatry, 157(7):1120-6.
Breslau, N., Davis, G.C., Andreski, P., Petersom, E.L., Schulz, L. 1997. Sex differences in posttraumatic stress disorder. Archives of General Psychiatry, 54: 81-87.

Brickman, J. 1984. Feminist, nonsexist, and traditional models of therapy: Implications for working with incest. Woman and Therapy, 3, 910, 49 – 67.

Briere, J. 1986. Suicidal thoughts and behaviours in former sexual abuse victims. Canadian Journal of Behavioural Science, Vol. 18(4), 413-423.

Briere J. 1998. Self-mutilation in clinical and general populations samples: Prevalence, correlates, and functions. American Journal of Orthopsychiatry, Vol. 68(4), 609-620.

—. 1992. Child abuse trauma. London: Sage.

—.2004. Psychological assessment of adult posttraumatic states: Phenomenology, diagnosis, and measurement. Washington, DC: American Psychological Association.

—. 2006a. Dissociative symptoms and trauma exposure: specificity, affect dysregulation, and posttraumatic stress. Journal of Nervous and Mental Disease, 194, 78-82.

Briere, J., Runtz, M. 1988. Multivariate correlates of childhood psychological and physical maltreatment among university women. Child Abuse and Neglect, 12, 331-341.

Briere, J. Scott, C. 2006. Principles of Trauma Therapy. A guide to symptoms, evaluation, and treatment. London: Sage.

Briere, J., Spinazzola, J. 2005. Phenomenology and Psychological Assessment of Complex Posttraumatic States. Journal of Traumatic Stress, Vol. 8, 5, 401-412.

Brodsky, B. S., Cloitre, M., Dulit, RA. 1995. Relationship of dissociation to self-mutilation and childhood abuse in borderline personality disorder. American Journal of Psychiatry, 152, 1788-1792.

Brown, D. 2009. Assessment of Attachment and Abuse History, and Adult Attachment Style. In Ch. Courtois, J. Ford, (Eds), Treating Complex Traumatic Stress Disorders. An Evidence - Based Guide (pp. 124-145). New York: The Guilford Press.

Brown, K., Herbert, M. 1999. Zapobieganie przemocy w rodzinie. [Prevention of domestic violence.]. Warszaw: PARPA.

Brownmiller, S. 1975. Against our will: Men, women and rape. New York: Simon and Schuster.

Bryant, R.A., Harley, A.G. 2000. Acute stress disorder: A handbook of theory, assessment, and treatment. Washington: APA.

Bryant, R. A., Gutrie, R. M. 2007. Maladaptive self-appraisals before trauma exposure predict posttraumatic stress disorder. Journal of Consulting and Clinical Psychology, Vol. 75(5), 812-815.

Brzezińska, A. 2003. Wydarzenia punktualne i niepunktualne w okresie dzieciństwa i dorastania. [Punctual and Unpunctual Events during the Childhood and Adolescence]. Remedium 130: 47-48.

Bremner, J., Krystal, J., Southwick, S., Charney, D. 1995. Functional neuroanatomical correlates of stress on memory. Journal of Traumatic Stress, 8 (4), 527-553.

Bremner, J., Scott, T., Delaney, R., Southwick, S., Mason, J., Johnson, D., Innis, R., McCarthy, G., Charney, D. 1993. Deficits in short – term memory in post – traumatic stress disorders. American Journal of Psychiatry, 150, 1015-1019.

Buss, A. H. 1962. The psychology of aggression. New York: Wiley.

Cabizuca, M., Marques-Portella, C., Mendlowicz, M .V., Coutinho, E.S., Figueira, I. 2009. Posttraumatic stress disorder in parents of children with chronic illness: A meta-analysis. Health Psychology, Vol. 28(3), 379-388.

Camarago, E. E. 2007. Brain SPECT in Neurology and Psychiatry, Journal of Nuclear Medicine, 2001, 42(4), 611-23.

Cameron, O. 2001. Interoception: the inside story - a model for psychosomatic processes. Psychosomatic Medicine, 63, 697-710.

Campbell, J.C. 2002. Health consequences of intimate partner violence. The Lancet, 359, 1331-1336.

Carlson, E.B., Putnam, F.W. 1993. An update on the Dissociative Experiences Scale. Dissociation, 6, 16-27.

Cassidy, J., Shaver, Ph. 1999. Handbook of Attachment. Theory, research, and Clinical Applications. London: The Guilford Press.

Chazan, B., Gabryś, M., Środoń, M., Wróblewska, W. 2007. Ekspertyza. Zdrowotne następstwa przedwczesnej inicjacji seksualnej u dziewcząt. [Expert's Report. Health Consequences of Girls' Early Sexual Initation].

Chrzanowska, J. 2005. Alienacja ofiar a stereotypy. [Alienacja ofiar a stereotypy]. Niebieska Linia nr 2/37, 6-8.

Chu, J. A. 1998. Rebuilding Shattered Lives: The Responsible Treatment of Complex Post-Traumatic and Dissociative Disorders. New York: John Wiley.

Cierpiałkowska, L. 2000. Alkoholizm. Przyczyny – leczenie – Profilaktyka. [Alcoholism. Causes - treatment - prevention.]. Poznań: UAM Scientific Publishing.

—. 2001. Psychoterapia psychoanalityczna i behawioralna pacjentów borderline. [Psychoanalytic psychotherapy and behavioral therapy of borderline patients.]. In L. Cierpiałkowska, H. Sęk (Eds.), Psychologia kliniczna i psychologia zdrowia [Clinical psychology and health psychology] (pp. 113-142). Poznań: Wydawnictwo Fundacji Humaniora.

—. 2002. Otto Kernberga psychoterapia skoncentrowana na przeniesieniu. [Otto Kernberg's psychotherapy focused on the transfer]. In L. Cierpiałkowska, J. Gościniak (Eds.), Współczesna psychoanaliza. Teorie relacji z obiektem. [Contemporary Psychoanalysis. Theories of object relations] (pp. 119-148). Poznań: Wydawnictwo Fundacji Humaniora.

—. 2006. Kierunki rozwoju współczesnej psychologii uzależnień (na przykładzie alkoholizmu). [Trends in the development of modern psychology of addiction (alcoholism as an example).]. In L. Cierpiałkowska (Ed.) Faces of modern addictions. Poznań: UAM Scientific Publishing.

—. 2007. Psychopatologia [Psychopathology]. Warszawa: Wydawnictwo Naukowe SCHOLAR.

Cioran, E. M. 2004. Księga złudzeń. [Book of illusions]. Warszawa: Wydawnictwo KR.

Cole, P., Putnam, F. 1992. Effect of incest on self and social functioning: A Developmental psychopathology perspective. Journal of Consulting and Clinical Psychology, 60: 174-184.

Collins, S., Long, A. 2003. Working with the psychological effects of trauma: consequences for mental healthcare workers - a literature review. Journal of Psychiatric and Mental Health Nursing, 10: 417-424.

Corrigan, F. M. 2004. Psychotherapy as assisted homeostasis: Activation of emotional processing mediated by the anterior cingulated cortex. Medical Hypothesis, 63: 968-973.

Courtois, Ch. 1998. Healing the incest wound. New York: Norton.

—. 2008. Complex trauma, complex reactions: Assessment and treatment. Psychological Trauma: Theory, Research, Practice, and Policy, Vol. S(1), 86-100.

—. 2009. The need for inclusion of psychological trauma in the Professional curriculum: A call to action. Psychological Trauma: Theory, Research, Practice, and Policy, Vol. 1 (1), 3-33.

Courtois, Ch., Ford, J. 2009. Treating Complex Traumatic Stress Disorders. An Evidence - Based Guide. New York: The Guilford Press.

Czapczyńska, M. 2007. Ochrona dzieci. Raport ONZ 2006. Niebieska Linia. [The protection of children. The UNO report, 2006. Blue Line.], 3, 32-34.

Darley, J.M., Bateson, C. D. 1973. From Jerusalem to Jericho: A study of situational and dispositional variables in helping behavior. Journal of Personality and Social Psychology, 27,1, 100-108.

Darley, J. M., Latane, B. 1968. Bystander intervention In emergencies: Diffusion of responsibility. Journal of Personality and Social Psychology, 8, 4, Pt.1, 377-383.
Daro, D., Cohn-Donnelly, A. C. 2004. Zapobieganie krzywdzeniu dzieci: osiągnięcia i wyzwania. Dziecko Krzywdzone. Teoria, badania, praktyka, 9, 1-19.
Davis, M., Whalen, P. J. 2001. The amygdala: vigilance and emotion. Molecular Psychiatry, 6:13-34.
Deighton, R. M., Gurris, N., Traue, H. 2007. Factors Affecting Burnout and Compassion Fatigue in Psychotherapists Treating Torture Survivors: Is the Therapist's Attitude to Working Through Trauma Relevant? Journal of Traumatic Stress, 20(1): 63-75.
Dell, P. F. 2006. The Multidimensional Inventory of dissociation (MID): a comprehensive measure of pathological dissociation. Journal of Trauma and Dissociation, 7, 77-106.
—. 2009. Understanding Dissociation. In P. F. Dell & JA O'Neil (Eds.), Dissociation and the Dissociative Disorders: DSM-V and Beyond (pp. 709-825). New York: Routledge.
Denzin, N. K. 1988. The Alcoholic Self. Newbury Park, Beverly Hills, London: SAGE Publications.
—. 2007. The Alcoholic Society: Addiction &Recovery of the Self. New Brunswick: Transaction Publishers.
Dębski, R. 1999. Ciąża i poród u młodocianych. Wychowanie seksualne i planowanie rodziny w Polsce. [Teenage Pregnancy and Delivery. Sexual Education and Family Planning in Poland.]. Warszawa: TRR.
Dobrzyńska-Mesterhazy, A. 1996. Przemoc w rodzinie: diagnoza i interwencja kryzysowa. [Domestic violence: diagnosis and crisis intervention.]. In W. Badura-Madej (Ed.), Wybrane zagadnienia interwencji kryzysowej. [Selected aspects of crisis intervention] (pp. 115-143). Warszawa: Interart.
Dolan, Y. 1991. Resolving sexual abuse. London: Norton & Company.
Donegan, N. H., Sanislow, C. A., Blumberg, H. P. 2003. Amygdala hyperreactivity in borderline personality disorder: implications for emotional dysregulation. Biological Psychiatry, 54, 1284-93.
Dovidio, L. F. 1984. Helping behavior and altruism: An empirical and conceptual overview. Advances in Experimental Social Psychology, 17, 361-427.
Draijer, N., Langeland, W. 1999. Childhood trauma and perceived parental dysfunction in the etiology of dissociative symptoms in psychiatric inpatients. American Journal of Psychiatry, 156, 379-385.

Dragon, M. 2008. Doświadczenia traumatyczne a uzależnienie od alkoholu. [Traumatic experiences and alcohol dependence.]. Warszawa: Wydawnictwo Uniwersytetu Warszawskiego.

Dudek, B. 2003. Zaburzenia po stresie traumatycznym. [Disorders after traumatic stress.]. Gdańsk: Gdańskie Wydawnictwo Psychologiczne.

Dutton, D. G. 1998. The Abusive Personality. Violence and Control in Intimate Relationships. London: The Guilford Press.

Dutton, D. 2003. Treatment of Assaultiveness. In D. Dutton, D. J. Sonkin (Eds.) Intimate Violence: Contemporary Treatment Innovations. New York: HMTP.

Dutton, M. R., Rubinstein, F. L. 1995. Working with people with PTSD: research implications. In R. C. Figley (Ed.), Compassion Fatigue: Coping with Secondary Traumatic Stress Disorder in Those Who Treat the Traumatized. (pp. 82-100). New York: Brunnar/Mazel.

Dyjakon, D. 2005. Przemoc i zadośćuczynienie. [Violence and gratification.]. Terapia Uzależnienia i Współuzależnienia, 5(44), 22-25.

—. 2006. Wpływ terapii na zmiany w relacjach rodzinnych alkoholików – sprawców przemocy domowej. [Influence of the psychotherapy on changes in relations of family alcoholics who perpetrate domestic violence.]. In J. Klebaniuk (Ed.), Człowiek wobec masowych zjawisk społecznych. Wrocław: Oficyna Wydawnicza ATUT.

—. 2007. The return of my dad. The world of problems, 1(168), 16-20.

—. 2010. Violence, therapy, gratification. Wrocław: DSW Publishing.

Ebner-Priemer, U. W., Badeck, S., Beckmann, C. 2005. Affective dysregulation and dissociative experience in female patients with borderline personality disorder: a startle response study. Journal of Psychiatric Research, 39, 85-92.

Elhai, J. D., Simons, J. S. 2007. Trauma exposure and posttraumatic stress disorder predictors of mental health treatment use in college students. Psychological Service, Vol. 4(1), 38-45.

Ellis, A. 1999. Jak opanować złość zanim ona opanuje ciebie. [How to Control Your Anger before it Controls You.]. Poznań: Media Rodzina.

—. 1999. Short-term therapy. Gdańsk: GWP.

Erikson, E. 1956. The problem of ego identity. American Journal of Psychoanalytic Association, 4: 56-118.

—. 1980. Identity and the Life Cycle. New York: W. W. Norton & Company.

Farrenkopf, T. 1992. What happens to therapists who work with sex offenders? Journal of Offender Rehabilitation, 18(3/4): 217-223.

Farrington, D. P. 2007. Family Background and Psychopathy. In Ch. J. Patrick, Handbook of Psychopathy (pp. 229-250). New York/London: The Guilford Press.

Fergusson, D. M., Horwood, L. J., Lynskey, M. T. 1997. Childhood sexual abuse, adolescent sexual behaviors and sexual revictimization. Child Abuse & Neglect: The International Journal, 21: 789-803.

Ferguson, G. F., Takane, Y. 2001. Analiza statystyczna w psychologii pedagogice. [Statistical analysis in psychology and pedagogy.]. Warszawa: PWN.

Figley, C. R. (Ed.), 1985. Trauma and its wake: The study and treatment of post-traumatic stress disorder. New York: Brunner/Mazel.

—. 1995. Compassion fatigue as secondary traumatic stress disorder: an overview. In C. R. Figley, Compassion Fatigue: Coping with Secondary Traumatic Stress Disorder in Those Who Treat the Traumatized (pp. 1-20). New York: Brunnar/Mazel.

Finkelhor, D. 1986. A sourcebook on child sexual abuse. Newbury Park, CA: Sage.

First, M.B., Spitzer, R.L., Gibbon, M., Williams, J. B. W. 1996. Structured Clinical Interview for DSM-IV Axis I Disorders, Clinician Version (SCID-CV). Washington, D.C.: American Psychiatric Press, Inc.

Fonagy, P., Gergely, G., Jurist, E., Target, M. 2002. Affect regulation, mentalization, and the development of self. New York: Other Press.

Ford, J., Courtois, Ch. 2009. Defining and Understanding Complex Trauma and Complex Traumatic Stress Disorders. In Courtois, Ch., Ford, J. (Eds). Treating Complex Traumatic Stress Disorders. An Evidence - Based Guide (pp. 13-31). New York: The Guilford Press.

Forgas, J. P., Wiliams K .D., Wheeler L. 2005. Umysł społeczny. Poznawcze i motywacyjne aspekty zachowań interpersonalnych. [The mind of society. Cognitive and motivational aspects of interpersonal behavior]. Gdańsk: Gdańskie Wydawnictwo Psychologiczne.

Freud, S. 1916/2000. Wstęp do psychoanalizy. [Introduction to Psychoanalysis.]. Warszawa: Wydawnictwo Naukowe PWN.

—. 1892/2001. O psychicznym mechanizmie zjawisk histerycznych.[The psychological mechanism of hysterical phenomena.]. In S. Freud, Histeria i lęk. [Hysteria and fear] (pp. 5-16). Warszawa: Wydawnictwo KR.

Frewen, P. A., Lanius, R. A. 2006. Neurobiology of dissociation: unity and disunity in mind-body-brain. Psychiatric Clinics of North America, 29, 113-128.

Friedman, M. 2001. Post Traumatic Stress Disorder. Kansas City: CC.

Frommberger, U. H., Stieglitz, R .D., Nyberg, E., Schlickewei, W., Kuner,

E. and Berger, M. 1998. Prediction of posttraumatic stress disorder by immediate reactions to trauma: a prospective study in road traffic accident victims. European Archives of Psychiatry and Clinical Neuroscience, 248(6): 316-21.

Fuchs, T. 2004. Neurobiology and psychotherapy: An emerging dialogue. Curr Opin Psychiatry, 17: 479-485.

Garland, C. 2009. Jak myśleć o traumie. [How to think about the trauma.]. In C. Garland, Czym jest trauma. Podejście psychoanalityczne. [What is trauma. Psychoanalytic approach.]. Warszawa: Oficyna Ingenium, 19-45.

Gessner, B. D., Perham-Hester, K. A. 1998. Experience of violence among teenage mothers in Alaska. Journal of Adolescent Health, 22: 383-388.

Gierowski, J.K., Heutzman, J., Rutkowski, K. 1996. Koncepcja sieci społecznej jako przykład nowoczesnego postępowania diagnostycznego w psychiatrii sądowej. [Conception of social network as a example of contemporary diagnostic procedure in forensic psychiatry.]. In J.K. Gierowski, A. Szymusik (Eds.), Postępowanie karne i cywilne wobec osób zaburzonych psychicznie. [Penal and civil procedure as aganist person with mentally diseased] (pp. 83-91). Kraków: Collegium Medicum UJ.

Gold, P. W. 2005. The neurobiology of stress and its relevance to psychotherapy. Clinical Neuroscience Research, 4: 315-324.

Golding, J. M. 1999. Intimate partner violence as risk factor for mental disorders: A meta-analysis. Journal of Family Violence, 1499-132.

Goodman, M., Weiss, D. S., Mitropoulou, V. 2003. The relationship between pathological dissociation, self-injury and childhood trauma in patients with personality disorders using taxometric analyses. Journal of Trauma and Dissociation, 4, 2, 65-88.

Gorski, T. T., Miller, M. 1991. Staying Sober. Jak wytrwać w trzeźwości. [A Guide for Relapse Prevention.]. Warszawa: Instytut Psychiatrii i Neurologii.

Graybar, S. R., Boutilier, L. R. 2002. Nontraumatic pathways to borderline personality disorder. Psychotherapy: Theory/ Research/ Practice/ Training 39 (2): 1,52-162.

Gregory, R. J., Chlebowski, S., Kang, D. 2008. A controlled trial of psychodynamic psychotherapy for co-occurring borderline personality disorder and alcohol use disorder. Psychotherapy: Theory, Research, Practice, Training, 45, 1, 28-41.

Gregurek, R. 1999. Countertransference problems in the treatment of a mixed group of war veterans and female partners of war veterans. Croatian Medical Journal, 40 (4): 493-497.

Grosjean, B. Tsai, G. E. 2007. NMDA neurotransmission as a critical mediator of borderline personality disorder. Journal of Psychiatry and Neuroscience, 32, 2, 102-115.

Gunderson, J. G. 1994. Borderline Personality Disorder. Washington, DC.: American Psychiatric Press.

Gunderson, J.G., Zanarini, M.C., Kisiel, C.L. 1991. Borderline personality disorder: a review of data on DSM-III-R descriptions. Journal of Personality Disorders, 5, 340-352.

Hamberger, L.K., Hastings, J. E. 1986. Personality correlates of men who abuse their partners: A cross validation study. Journal of Family Violence, 1, 323-341.

Hamilton-Giachritsis, C., Browne, K., Falshaw, L. 2005. Krzywdzenie dzieci w rodzinie i poza rodziną oraz jego związek z zachowaniami przestępczymi dzieci. Dziecko Krzywdzone, 10, 79 - 92 .

Hamilton, C. E., Browne, K. D. 1998. The repeat victimisation of children: should the concept be revised? Aggression and Violent Behaviour, 3(1): 47-60.

Hammond, W. R., Haegerich T. M., Saul, J. 2009. Psychological Service, 6, 4, 3, 253-263.

Hare, R. D. 1991/2002. The Hare Psychopathy Checklist-Revised. Toronto, ON: Multi-Health Systems.

Harned, M. 2000. Harassed bodies: An examination of the relationships among women's experiences of sexual harassment, body image and eating disturbances. Psychology of Women Quarterly, 24: 336-348.

Hebrang, A., Henigsberg, N. and Hrabac, P. 2006. Evacuation times of civilians and soldiers wounded during the war in Croatia. Military Medicine, 171 (11): 1045-1050.

Hebrang, A., Henigsberg, N., Golem, A.Z., Vidjak, V., Brnic, Z., Hrabac, P. 2006. Care of military and civilian casualties during the war in Croatia. Acta Medica Croatica, 60 (4): 301-137.

Heim, C., Plotsky, P.M., Nemeroff, C.B. 2004. Importance of studying the contributions of early adverse experience to neurobiological findings in depression. Neuropsychopharmacology, 29: 641-648.

Heilbrun, A., Orr, H., Harrell, S. 1966. Patterns of parental childrearing and consequent vulnerability to cognitive disturbance. Journal of Consult. Psychology, 30, 51 – 59.

Herman, J. 1998, 2003. Uraz i powrót do równowagi. [Trauma and recovery.]. Gdańsk: Gdańskie Wydawnictwo Psychologiczne.

—. 1992. Trauma and Recovery. New York: BasicBooks.

—. 1992a. Complex PTSD: A syndrome in survivors of prolonged and repeated trauma. Journal of Traumatic Stress, 5, 377-39.

Herman, J., Perry, J., van der Kolk, B. 1989. Childhood trauma in borderline personality disorder. American Journal of Psychiatry, 22, 231-237.

Herman, J., Van der Kolk, B. 1987. Traumatic antecedents of borderline personality disorder. In B. Van der Kolk (Ed.), Psychological trauma (pp. 111-126). Washington, DC: American Psychiatric Press.

Hamberger, L. K., Hastings, J. E. 1986. Personality correlates of men who abuse their partners: A cross validation study. Journal of Family Violence, 1, 323-341.

Herzberger, S. D. 2002. Przemoc domowa - perspektywa psychologii społecznej. [Domestic violence - the prospect of social psychology.]. Warszawa: Państwowa Agencja Rozwiązywania Problemów Alkoholowych.

—. 2003. Rola stereotypów w diagnozowaniu przemocy. [The role of stereotypes in the diagnosis of violence.]. Niebieska Linia nr 1, http: //www.pismo.niebieskalinia.pl/index.php

Hidalgo, R. B., Davidson, J. R. T. 2000. Post-traumatic stress disorder: Epidemiology and health-related considerations. Journal of Clinical Psychiatry, 61 (Supplement 7), 5-13.

Hillis, S. D., Anda, R. F., Dube, S.R., Felitti, V.J., Marchbanks, P. A., Marks, J.S. 2004. The association between adverse childhood experiences and adolescent pregnancy, long-term psychosocial consequences, and fetal death. Pediatrics, 113: 320-327.

Hodalic, Z., Svagelj, M., Sebalj, I., Sebalj, D. 1999. Surgical treatment of 1, 211 patients at the Vinkovci General Hospital, Vinkovci, Croatia, during the 1991-1992 Serbian offensive in east Slavonia. Military Medicine, 164 (11): 803-808.

Hoffman, M. L. 2006. Empatia i rozwój moralny. [Empathy and moral development.]. Gdańsk: Gdańskie Wydawnictwo Psychologiczne.

Holmes, E. A., Brown, R .J., Mansell, W., Fearon, R. P., Hunter, E .C. 2005. Are there two qualitatively distinct forms of dissociation? A review and some clinical implication. Clinical Psychology Review, 25 (1): 1023.

Hołyst, B. 1999. Kryminologia. [Criminology.]. Warszawa: PWN, sixth enlarged edition.

Howe, A. C., Herzberger S. D., Tennen H. 1988. The influence of personal history of abuse and gender on clinicians' judgments of child abuse. Journal of Family Violence, 3(2), 105-119.

International Society for Study of Dissociation. 2005. Guidelines for treating dissociative identity disorder. Journal of Trauma and Dissociation, 6, 69-149.

ICD - 10. 1998. Classification of psychological disorders and behaviour disorders in ICD - 10. Research diagnostic criteria. Kraków: Medical University Publishing.

ICD - 10. 2000. International Statistical Classification of Diseases and Health problems . Kraków: Medical University Publishing.

Iwon, A. 2009. Radny PiS: Ciężarne uczennice trzeba izolować od innych uczniów [Law and Justice's Councillor: The Pregnant Schoolgirls Should be Isolated from Other Pupils]. http://www.mmpulawy.pl/artykul/radny-pis-ciezarne-uczennice-trzeba-izolowac-od-innych-czniow-34211.html. (accessed September 12, 2009).

Jang, K. L., Livesley, W. J., Ver non, P. A., Jackson, D.N. 1996. Heritability of personality disorder traits: a twin study. Acta Psychiatrica Scandinavica, 94, 438-444.

Juczynski, Z., Ogińska-Bulik, N. 2009. Pomiar zaburzeń po stresie traumatycznym - polska wersja Zrewidowanej Skali Wpływu Zdarzeń. [Measurement traumatic stress disorder - a Polish version of the Revised Impact of Event Scale.]. Psychiatria, 6 (1): 15-25

Judd, P. H. 2005. Neurocognitive impairment as a moderator in the development of borderline personality disorder. Development and Psychopathology, 17, 1173-1196.

Juni, J. E., Waxman, A. D., Devous, M. D., Tikofsky, R .S., Ichise, M., Van Heertum, R.L., Holman, B.L., Carretta, R.F. and Chen, C.C. 1998. Procedure guideline for brain perfusion SPECT using technetium-99m radiopharmaceuticals. Journal of Nuclear Medicine, 39 (5): 923-6.

Kadambi, M.A., Truscott, D. 2004. Vicarious trauma among therapists working with sexual violence, cancer, and general practice. Canadian Journal of Counseling, (38): 260-276.

Kandel, E.R. 1999. Biology and the future of psychoanalysis: A new intellectual framework for psychiatry research. American Journal of Psychiatry, 156: 505-524.

Kassam-Adams, N. 1995. The risks of treating sexual trauma: Stress and secondary trauma in psychotherapists. In B. H. Stamm (Ed.), Secondary traumatic stress: Self-care issues for clinicians, researchers and educators. (pp. 37-48). 2nd edition. Lutherville, MD: Sidran Press.

Kazdin, A. E. 2009. Bridging science and practice to improve patent care. American Psychologist, Vol. 64 (4), 276-279.

Kiser, L.J., Heston, J., Millsap, P.A., Pruitt, D.B. 1991. Physical and sexual abuse in childhood: Relationship with post-traumatic stress disorders. Journal of the American Academy of Child and Adolescent Psychiatry, 30 (5): 776-783.

Kellogg, N.D., Hoffman, T.J., Taylor, E.R. 1999. Early sexual experiences among pregnant and parenting adolescents, Adolescence, 34: 293-303.

Kendall-Tackett, K. 2009. Psychological trauma and physical health: A psychoneuroimmunology approach to etiology of negative health effects and possible interventions. Psychological Trauma: Theory, Research, Practice, and Policy, Vol. 1(1), 35-48.

Kernberg, O. F. 1976. Object-relations theory and clinical psychoanalysis. New York: Jason Aronson Inc.

—. 1980. Psychotherapy with borderline patients: An overview. In B. Karasu, L. Bellak (Eds.), Specialized techniques for specific clinical problems in psychotherapy (pp. 85-117). Northvale, New Jersey, London: Jason Aronson Inc.

—. 1996. A psychoanalytic theory of personality disorders. In J. F. Clarkin and M. F. Lenzenweger (Eds.), Major theories of personality disorders (pp. 106-140). New York London: The Guilford Press.

—. 2004. Borderline personality disorder and borderline personality organization: Psychopathology and psychotherapy. In J. J. Magnavita (Ed.), Handbook of personality disorders (pp. 92-119). New Jersey: John Wiley & Sons, Inc.

Kessler, R.C., Sonnega, A., Bromet, E, Hughes, M, Nelson, C.B. 1995. Posttraumatic stress disorder in the National Comorbidity Survey. Archives of General Psychiatry, 55, 801-800.

Koehn, C. 2007. Women's Perceptions of Power and Control in Sexual Abuse Counseling. Child sexual abuse, Vol. 16, 1, 37 – 61.

Koons, C. R., Robins, C.J., Tweed, J. L. et al. 2001. Efficacy of dialectical behaviour therapy in women veterans with borderline personality disorder. Behavior Therapy, 32: 371-390.

Korkeila, J., Lehtinen, V., Bijl, R., Dalgard, O-S., Kovess, V. 2003. Establishing a set of mental health indicators for Europe. Scandinavica Journal of Public Health, 31(6): 451-459.

Korzekwa, M. I. Dell, P. F. Links, P. S. Thabane, L. Fougere, P. 2009. Dissociation in Borderline Personality Disorder: A Detailed Look. Journal of Trauma & Dissociation, 10, 346-367.

Korzekwa, M.I., Dell, P.F., Links, P.S., Thabane, L., Webb, S.P. 2008. Estimating the prevalence of borderline personality disorder in psychiatric outpatients using a two-phase procedure. Comprehensive Psychiatry, 49, 380-386.

Korzekwa, M.I., Dell, P.F., Pain, C. 2009. Dissociation and Borderline Personality Disorder: An Update for Clinicians. Current Psychiatry Reports, 11, 82-88.

Kościelska, M. 1998. Trudne macierzyństwo. [The Difficult Motherhood]. Warszawa: Wydawnictwa Szkolne i Pedagogiczne.

Kowalik, S. 2003. Ja cielesne-próba nowego spojrzenia. [The physical self- an attempt at new approach.]. Polskie Forum Psychologiczne, 1: 5-29.

Koyama, M., Kawashima, R., Ito, H., Ono, S., Sato, K., Goto, R., Kinomura, S., Yoshioka, S., Sato, T. and Fukuda, H. 1997. SPECT imaging of normal subjects with technetium-99m-HMPAO and technetium-99m-ECD. Journal of Nuclear Medicine, 38(4):587-92.

Kozłowska, A. 1998. Wpływ czynników biologicznych i psychicznych na czucie dotyku u dzieci. Niepublikowana praca doktorska. [Influence of biological and psychic factors on touch threshold among children]. Unpublished doctoral dissertation, University of Adam Mickiewicz, Poland.

Kraus, V. 2005. Relationship Between Self-Care and Compassion Satisfaction, Compassion Fatigue, and Burnout Among Mental Health Professionals Working with Adolescent Sex Offenders. Counseling and Clinical Psychology Journal 2 (1): 81-88.

Kremers, I.P., Spinoven, P., Van der Does, A.J.W., Van Dyck, R. 2006. Autobiographical memory in depressed and nondepressed patients with borderline personality disorder after long-term psychotherapy. Cognition and Emotion, 20, 3/4, 448-465.

Krueger, D. 2002. Integrating body self and psychological self. New York, London: Brunner-Routledge.

Kuczyńska, A. 2009. Stres traumatyczny. [Traumatic stress]. Referat wygłoszony na I Międzynarodowej Konferencji Naukowej pt." Zrozumienie Interpersonalnej Traumy - mechanizmy i konsekwencje w rodzinie i środowisku. Teoria i praktyka.". [A paper presented at the First International Scientific Conference. "Understanding Interpersonal Trauma - mechanisms and consequences in the family and the environment. Theory and practice."]. Wrocław (nonpublic material).

Kubacka-Jasiecka. 2004. Nie widzę, nie słyszę i milczę...O psychologii świadków przemocy. [I don't see, don't hear and I keep silent ... The psychology of witnesses of violence.]. In P. Piotrowski (Ed.), Przemoc i marginalizacja. Patologia społecznego dyskursu. [Violence and marginalization. Pathology of social discourse]. (pp. 183- 221). Warszawa: Wydawnictwo Akademickie „Żak".

Kurza, K. 2004. Na kłopoty kurator. [For trouble curator.]. Niebieska Linia, 4, 20- 22.

Kurza, K. 2005. Za zamkniętym drzwiami. [Behind closed door]. Niebieska Linia, 1, 22-25.

Laddis, A., Dell, PF. 2002. A comparison of DID with 30 cases of SIDP-IV diagnosed borderline personality disorder. Presented at the 19th

annual meeting of the International Society for the Study of Dissociation. Baltimore, USA.
Landry, D. J., Forrest J. D. 1995. „How old are US fathers?" Family Planning Perspectives, 27: 159-161.
Lange, C., Kracht, L., Herholz, K., Sachsse, U., Irle, E. 2005. Reduced glucose metabolism in temporo-parietal cortices of women with borderline personality disorder. Psychiatry Research: Neuroimaging, 139, 115-126.
Lang, P.J., Bradley, M.M., Cuthbert, B.N. 1998. Emotion, Motivation, and Anxiety: Brain Mechanisms and Psychophysiology, Biological Psychiatry, 44:1248-1263.
Lanius, R.A., Williamson, P.C., Bluhm, R.L., et al. 2005. Functional connectivity of dissociative responses in posttraumatic stress disorder: a functional magnetic resonance imaging investigation. Biological Psychiatry, 57, 873-884.
Lansen, J. 2001. What does this work do to us? In S. Graessner, N. Gurris and C. Pross (Eds.), At the side of torture survivors: Treating a terrible assault on human dignity (pp. 198-211). Baltimore, MD: Johns Hopkins University Press.
Laplanche, J., Pontalis, J.-B. 1996. Słownik psychoanalizy. [Dictionary of psychoanalysis.]. Warszawa: Wydawnictwo Szkolne i Pedagogiczne.
Laporte, L., Guttman, H. 2001. Abusive relationships in families of women with borderline personality disorder, anorexia nervosa, and a control group. Journal of Nervous and Mental Disease, 189, 522-531.
Latane, B., Darley, J. M. 1968. Group inhibition of bystander intervention in emergencies. Journal of Personality and Social Psychology, 10, 215-221.
Latane, B., Darley, J. M. 1970. The unresponsive bystander: Why doesn't he help? New York: Appleton-Century Crofts.
Lawson D. M., Brossart D. F. 2009. Attachment, interpersonal problem, and treatment outcome in group therapy for intimate partner violence. Psychology Man and Masculinity, 10, 4, 288-301.
Le Doux, J. 1986. Mind and brain: dialogues in cognitive neuro-science, New York: Cambridge University Press.
Leiderman, S., Almo, C. 2001. Interpersonal violence and adolescent pregnancy: Prevalence and implications for practice and policy. Washington, DC: Healthy Teen Network.
Leonard. K., Blane, T. 2003. Picie i alkoholizm w świetle teorii psychologicznych. [Psychological Theories of Drinking and Alcoholism.]. Wraszawa: Państwowa Agencja Rozwiązywania Problemów Alkoholowych.

Leszczyńska A., Benight C.C., Cieślak R. 2009. Self-efficacy and heath-related outcomes of collective trauma: A systematic review. European Psychologist, Vol. 14(1), 51-62.

Lew-Starowicz, Z. 2000. Forensic Sexology. Warsaw: PZWL.

Levine, P. 2005. Healing Trauma. A pioneering Program for Restoring the wisdom of Your Body. Sounds True.

Liberzon, I., Taylor, S.F., Amdur, R., Jung, T.D., Chamberlain, K.R., Minoshima, S., Koeppe, R.A., Fig, L.M. 1999. Brain activation in PTSD in response to trauma-related stimuli. Biological Psychiatry, 45(7): 817-26.

Linehan, M.M. 1987. Dialectical behavior therapy for borderline personality disorder. Theory and method. Bulletin of the Menninger Źlinic, 51 (3): 261-276.

—. 2007. Zaburzenie osobowości z pogranicza. Terapia poznawczo-behawioralna. [Borderline personality disorder. Cognitive-behavioral therapy.]. Kraków: Wydawnictwo Uniwersytetu Jagiellońskiego.

Links, P.S., Steiner, M., Offord, D.R. et al. 1988. Characteristics of borderline personality disorder: a Canadian study. Canadian Journal of Psychiatry, 33, 336-340.

Linley, P.A., Joseph, S. 2007. Therapy Work and Therapist's Positive and Negative Well-being. Journal of Social and Clinical Psychology, 26(3): 385-403.

Liotti, G. 2002. The inner schema of borderline states and its correction during psychotherapy: a cognitive-evolutionary approach. Journal of Cognitive Psychotherapy, 16, 3, 349-366.

Lis-Turlejska, M. 1998. Traumatyczny stres: Koncepcje i badania. [Traumatic stress: concepts and survey.]. Warszawa: Wydawnictwo Instytutu Psychologii PAN.

—. 2002. Stres traumatyczny. Występowanie, następstwa, terapia. [Traumatic stress. Occurrence, consequences, treatment.]. Warszaw: Wydawnictwo Akademickie "Żak".

—. 2005. Traumatyczne zdarzenia i ich skutki psychiczne. [Traumatic events and their psychological effects.. Warszawa: Wydawnictwo Instytutu Psychologii PAN.

Logan, C., Holcombe, E., Ryan, S., Manlove, J., Moore, K. 2007. Childhood sexual abuse and teen pregnancy. Child Trends Inc. http://www.thenationalcampaign.org. (accessed August 20, 2009).

Loncar, M., Medved, V., Jovanovic, N., Hotujac, L. 2006. Psychological consequences of rape on women in 1991-1995 war in Croatia and Bosnia and Herzegovina. Croatian Medical Journal, 47(1): 67-75.

Löffler-Stastka, H., Szerencsics, M., Blüml, V. 2009. Dissociation, trauma, affect regulation and personality in patients with a borderline personality organization. Bulletin of the Menninger Clinic, 73(2): 81-98.

Lykken, D.T. 2003. The Case for Parental Licensure. In T. Millon, E. Simonsen, M. Birket-Smith, R.D. Davie (Eds.), Psychopathy. Antisocial, Criminal and Violent Behavior (pp. 122-143). New York/London: The Guilford Press.

Mac, A. 2005. Wczesne dzieciństwo młodocianych przestępców agresywnych. [Early childhood of violent juvenile offenders.]. Poznań: Oficyna Wydawnicza GARMOND.

Maes, M., Mylle, J., Delmeire, L., Altamura, C. 2000. Psychiatric morbidity and comorbidity following accidental man-made traumatic events: incidence and risk factors. European Archives of Psychiatry and Clinical Neuroscience, 250(3): 156-62.

Magnavita, J.J. 2004. Classification, prevalence, and etiology of personality disorders: Related issues and controversy. In J. J. Magnavita (Ed.), Handbook of personality disorders (pp. 3-23). New Jersey: John Wiley & Sons, Inc.

Main, M., Hesse, E. 1990. Parents' unresolved traumatic experiences are related to infant disorganized attachment status: is frightened and/or frightening parental behaviour the linking mechanism? In M.T. Greenberg, D. Cicchetti, E.M. Cummings (Eds.), Attachment in the preschool years (pp. 161-182). Chicago: University Press of Chicago.

Malicka, M. 2003. Ciąże nastolatek - przyczyny, skutki, statystyki. Broszura informacyjna Federacji na rzecz Kobiet i Planowania Rodziny. [Teen Pregnancies-Causes, Effects, Statistics. Leaflet of Polish Federation for Women and Family Planning.]. http://www.federa.org.pl/publikacje/mat_info/ciazenast.htm. (accessed September 2, 2009).

Martens, W.H.J. 2005. Multimodal model of trauma and correlated antisocial personality disorders. Journal of Loss & Trauma, 10(2): 115-129.

Masten, A.S., Roisman, G.I., Long, J.D., Burt, K.B., Obradović, J. 2005. Developmental cascades: Linking academic achievement and externalizing and internalizing symptoms over 20 years. Developmental Psychology, 41(5): 733-746.

Mazur, J. 2002. Przemoc w rodzinie. [Domestic violence]. Warszawa: Wyd. Nauk. Żak

McDermott, I., Jago, W. 2006. Brie NLP Therapy. Sopot: GWP.

Mc Kay, A. 2006. Trends in teen pregnancy in Canada with comparisons to U.S.A. and England/Wales. The Canadian Journal of Human Sexuality, 15: 157-161.

Mellibruda, J. 1995. The trap of unforgiven harm. Warszawa: The Institute of Psychology, Health and Sobriety.

Mellibruda, J. 1997. Psycho-bio-social model of alcohol dependence. Alcohol and drug addiction, 3,28, 277-306.

Mellibruda, J. 1999. Psychological conception of the mechanisms of addiction. The Therapy of Addiction and Co-addition (1).

Mellibruda, J., Sobolewska-Mellibruda, Z. 2006. Integrating psychotherapy of addictions. Theory and practice. Warszawa: The Institute of Health Psychology.

Messman, T. L., Long, P. J. 1996. Child sexual abuse and its relationship to revictimization in adult women. A review. Clinical Psychology Review, 16: 397-420.

Miller, T.W. 2007. Trauma, change, and psychological health in the 21st century. American Psychologist, Vol. 62(8), 889-898.

Mirucka, B. 2003. Ja cielesne fundamentem tożsamości. [Physical self as a personality basis.]. Polskie Forum Psychologiczne, 8: 30-40.

Mirzaei, S., Knoll, P., Keck, A., Preitler, B., Gutierrez, E., Umek, H., Kohn, H. and Pecherstorfer, M. 2001, Regional cerebral blood flow in patients suffering from post-traumatic stress disorder, Neuropsychobiology, 43(4): 260-4.

Morgan, A.H. 1973. The heritability of hypnotic susceptibility of twins. Journal of Abnormal Psychology, 82, 55-61.

Muehlenhard, Ch. L., Peterson, Z. D. 2008. Konceptualizacja przemocy seksualnej. Przymus posiadający społeczne przyzwolenie i inne kontrowersje. [Conceptualization of sexual violence. Coercion socially acceptable and other controversies.]. In A. G. Miller (Ed.), Dobro i zło z perspektywy psychologii społecznej. [Good and evil from the perspective of social psychology.]. (pp. 304-338). Warszawa: Wydawnictwo WAM.

Mussgay, L., Klinkenberg, N., Rüddel, H. 1999. Heart beat perception in patients with depressive, somatoform, and personality disorders. Journal of Psychophysiology, 13: 27-36.

Niehoff, D. 2001. Biologia przemocy. Jak zrozumienie mózgu, zachowania i środowiska może przerwać błędne koło przemocy. [The Biology of Violence. How Understanding the Brain, Behavior, and Environment Can Break the Vicious Circle of Aggression.]. Poznań; Media Rodzina.

Nijenhuis, E., Spinhoven, P., van Dyck, R., van der Hart, O., Vanderlinden,

J. 1998. Degree of somatoform and psychological dissociation in dissociative disorder is correlated with reported trauma. Journal of Traumatic Stress, 11: 711-730.

Nikodemska, S. 2002. W służbie dzieciom. Przemoc wobec dzieci - opinie i postawy służb i instytucji społecznych w gminie. Warszawa Włochy. [In the service of children. Violence against children - opinions and attitudes of social services and institutions in the municipality of Warsaw Włochy.]. Niebieska Linia, 2, 30-33.

Noll, J.G., Trickett, P.K., Putnam, F.W. 2003. A Prospective investigation of the impact of childhood sexual abuse on the development of sexuality. Journal of Consulting and Clinical Psychology, 71: 575-586.

Norris, F.H., Murphy, A.D., Baker, C.K., Perilla, J.L., Rodriguez, Rodriguez, F.G. 2003. Epidemiology of trauma and posttraumatic stress disorder in Mexico. Journal of Abnormal Psychology, 112, 646-656.

Nowakowska, U., Jabłońska, M. 1998. Przemoc wobec kobiet. In Kobiety w Polsce w latach dziewięćdziesiątych. Raport Centrum Praw Kobiet. [Violence against women. In: Women in Poland in the nineties. Report Women's Rights Center.]. http://temida.free.ngo.pl/raport.htm

Nowakowska, U., Jabłońska, M. 2003. Przemoc wobec kobiet. [Violence against Women.]. In U. Nowakowska (Ed.), Kobiety w Polsce. Raport Centrum Praw Kobiet. [Women in Poland. Report of Women's Rights Center] (pp. 159-198). Warszawa: Centrum Praw Kobiet.

Nowakowska, B., Paluch, E., Zarębińska – Szczodry, E. 2001. Dzieciństwo bez przemocy. Rola Ośrodków Pomocy Społecznej we wspieraniu osób uzależnionych i ofiar przemocy. [Childhood without violence. In: The Role of Social Welfare Centres in helping drug addicts and victims of violence. X National Conference of the Association of Municipal Social Welfare Centres "Forum"]. X Ogólnopolska Konferencja Stowarzyszenia Samorządowych Ośrodków Pomocy Społecznej „Forum", Olsztyn.

Nowicka, W., (Ed.), 2007. Prawa reprodukcyjne w Polsce. Skutki ustawy antyaborcyjnej. Raport [Reproductive Rights in Poland. Consequences of Antiabortion Act. Report.]. http://www.federa.org.pl/index.php?page=article&catid=854&lang=1. (accessed September 1, 2009).

O'Farrell, T. J. 1999. Behavioral Couples Therapy for Alcoholism and Drug Abuse. Psychiatric Times, Vol. XVI, Issue 4.

O'Farrell, T. J., Murphy, C.M. 1995. Marital violence before and after alcoholism treatment. Journal of Consulting & Clinical Psychology, 63, 256-262.

O'Farrell, T. J., Van Hutton, V., Murphy, C.M. 1999. Domestic Violence before and Treatment: A Two-Year Longitudinal Study. Journal of Studies on Alcohol , 60, 3, 317-321.

OBOS-Ośrodek Badania Opinii Publicznej. 2007. Potrzeby szkoleniowe grup zawodowych „pierwszego kontaktu" z przypadkami przemocy w rodzinie. Wyniki badań TNS OBOP dla Ministerstwa Pracy i Polityki Społecznej. [OBOS-Center for Public Opinion Research. 2007. Training needs of professional "first contact" groups with cases of domestic violence. The results of TNS OBOP for the Ministry of Labour and Social Policy.]. Warszawa, www.tns-global.pl.

Obuchowska, I. 1989. Przemoc w Wychowaniu. [Violence in upbringing.]. Kwartalnik Pedagogiczny, 4, 27-41.

Obuchowski, K. 2000. Człowiek intencjonalny, czyli o tym, jak być sobą. [Man intentional, or about how to be ourselves.]. Poznań: Dom Wydawniczy REBIS.

Odgers, C.L., Reppucci, N.D., Morett, M.M. 2005. Nipping psychopathy in the bud: An examination of the convergent, predictive, and theoretical utility of the PCL-YV among adolescent girls. Behawioral Sciences and the Law, 23, 743-763.

Ogawa, J.R., Sroufe, L.A., Weinfield, N.S. et al. 1997. Development and the fragmented self: longitudinal study of dissociative symptomatology in a nonclinical sample. Development and Psychopathology, 9, 855-879.

Ogden, P., Minton, K., Pain, C. 2006. Trauma and the body. A sensorimotor Approach to Psychotherapy. London: W.W. Norton & Company.

Oltmanns, T.F., Emery, R.E. 2007. Abnormal Psychology. New Jersey: Pearson Education Inc.

Orbach, I., Mikulincer, M., King, R., Cohen D., Stein, D. 1997. Thresholds and tolerance of physical pain in suicidal and nonsuicidal adolescents. Journal of Consulting and Clinical Psychology, 65: 646-652.

Osipczuk, www.e-lama.pl

Ostrowska, K. 1981. Psychologiczne determinanty przestępczości młodocianych [Psychological determinants of juvenile delinquency.]. Warszawa: PWN.

Ozer, E.J., Best, S.R., Lipsey, T.L., Weiss, D.S. 2003. Predictors of posttraumatic stress disorder and symptoms in adults: A meta-analysis. Psychological Bulletin, Vol. 129(1), 52-73.

Paris, J., Zweig-Frank, H. 2001. A 27-year follow-up of patients with borderline personality disorder. Comprehensive Psychiatry, 42, 482-487.

Parkes, M., Stevenson – Hinde, J., Marris, P. 1993. Across the Life Cycle. New York: Routledge.

Pastwa-Wojciechowska, B. 2004. Naruszanie norm prawnych w psychopatii. Analiza kryminologiczno-psychologiczna. [Violations of legal norms in psychopathy. Criminological and psychological analysis.]. Gdańsk: Wydawnictwo UG.

—. 2010. Doświadczenia wczesnodziecięce osób o psychopatycznej strukturze osobowości: Retrospektywne badania czynników rodzinnych i społecznych. [Early childhood experiences of people with psychopathic personality structure: A retrospective study of family and social factors.], In T. Rostowska and A. Jarmołowska (Eds.), Rozwojowe i wychowawcze aspekty życia rodzinnego. [Developmental and educational aspects of family life.] (pp. 65-80). Warszawa: Difin.

Patton, M. 1990. Qualitative Evaluation and Research Methods. London: Sage Pbl.

Pearlman, L. 1998. Trauma and the self: A theoretical and clinical perspective. Journal of Emotional Abuse, 1, 7-25.

—. 2003. Trauma and Attachment Belief Scale. Los Angeles: Western Psychological Services.

Pearlman, L.A., Courtois, Ch. 2005. Clinical Applications of the Attachment Framework: Relational Treatment of Complex Trauma. Journal of Traumatic Stress, Vol. 18, 5, 449-461.

Pearlman, L.A., Saakvitne, P.S. 1995. Vicarious traumatization: An empirical study of the effects of trauma work on trauma therapists. Professional Psychology: Research and Practice, (26): 558-565.

Pelcovitz, D., Van der Kolk, B., Roth, S., Mandel, F., Kaplan, S., Resick, P. 1997. Development of a criteria set and a structured interview for disorders of extreme stress (DESNOS). Journal of Traumatic Stress, 10, 3 - 16.

Perris, C., Arrindell, W., Eisemann, M. 1994. Parenting and Psychopathology. New York: Wiley.

Perron, B.E., B.S. Hiltz. 2006. Burnout and Secondary Trauma Among Forensic Interviewers of Abused Children. Child and Adolescent Social Work Journal, 23(2): 216-234.

Perry, B.D., Pollard, B.A., Blakley, T.L., Baker, W.L., Vigilante, D. 1995. Childhood trauma, the neurobiology of adaptation and "use-dependent" development of the brain. Infant Mental Health Journal, 16, 4, 271-291.

Philipsen, A., Schmahl, C., Lieb, K. 2004. Naloxone in the treatment of acute dissociative states in female patients with borderline personality disorder. Pharmacopsychiatry, 37, 196-199.

Piliavin, J.A., Dovidio, J.R, Gaertner, S.L., Clark, R.D., III. 1981. Emergency intervention. New York: Academic Press.

Pissiota, A., Frans, O., Fernandez, M., Von Knorring, L., Fischer, H. and Fredrikson, M. 2002. Neurofunctional correlates of posttraumatic stress disorder: a PET symptom provocation study. European Archives of Psychiatry and Clinical Neuroscience, 252(2): 68-75.

Polish Federation for Women and Family Planning. 2008. Po wakacjach bez zmian. Edukacja seksualna po polsku. Informacja prasowa, czerwiec 2008. [No Changes after Holidays. Polish Sexual Education. Press release, June 2008]. http://www.federa.org.pl/page=article&catid =859&lang=1. (accessed September 1, 2009).

—. 2009. Porozumienie na rzecz upowszechniania edukacji seksualnej. Edukacja seksualna do szkół. Informacja prasowa, 20 stycznia 2009. [The Agreement for the Benefit of Sexual Education's Popularization. It's Time to Sexual Education at School. Press release, January 20, 2009.]. http://www.federa.org.pl/?page=news&newsid=597&lang=1. (accessed September 1, 2009).

Polish Ministry of Health. Raport: Zdrowie kobiet w wieku prokreacyjnym 15-49 lat. Polska 2006. [Report: Health fo Women in Procreative Age 15-49. Poland 2006.]. http://www.mz.gov.pl/wwwmz/index(accessed September 2, 2009).

Pospiszyl, I. 1994, 1998. Przemoc w rodzinie. [Violence in the family.]. Warszawa: WsiP.

—. 2003. Ofiary chroniczne. Przypadek czy konieczność. [Victims of chronic. Chance or necessity.]. Warszawa: Wydawnictwo Akademii Pedagogiki Specjalnej.

Pretzer, J.L., Beck, A.T. 1996. A cognitive theory of personality disorders. In J.F. Clarkin and M.F. Lenzenweger (Eds.), Major theories of personality disorders (pp. 36-105). New York, London: The Guilford Press.

Putnam, F. 1997. Dissociation in children and adolescents. A developmental perspective. New York: The Guilford Press.

Raine, A. Sanmartin, J. 2001. Violence and Psychopathy. New York: Academic Press.

Rainey, D.Y., Stevens-Simon, C., Kaplan, D. W. 1995. Are adolescents who report prior sexual abuse at higher risk for pregnancy? Child Abuse & Neglect, 19: 1283-1288.

Rada Ministrów RP. 2009. Sprawozdanie z wykonania ustawy o planowaniu rodziny, ochronie płodu ludzkiego i warunkach dopuszczalności przerywania ciąży w 2007 roku. [Report of on the Implementation of the Family Planning, Preservation of Human

Foetus, and the Conditions of Admissibility of Abortion, and the Consequences of its Performance Act in 2007.]. http://sejmometr.pl/raport/wmnCv. (accessed September 2, 2009).

Radke-Yarrow, M. 1993. Attachmant patterns in children of depressed mothers. In Parkes, M., Stevenson – Hinde, J., Marris, P. (Eds.), Across theLife Cycle (pp. 115-127). New York: Routledge.

Read, J., VanOs, J., Morrison, A.P., Ross, C.A. 2005. Childhood trauma, psychosis and schizophrenia: a literature review with theoretical and clinical implications. Acta of Psychiatrica Scandinavica, 112(5): 330-350.

Reinders, A.A., Nijenhuis, ERS., Quak, J., et al. 2006. Psychobiological characteristics of dissociative identity disorder: a symptom provocation study. Biological Psychiatry, 60, 730-740.

Reykowski, J. 1979. Motywacja, postawy prospołeczne a osobowość. [Motivation, attitudes and prosocial personalisty.]. Warszawa: PWN.

Riahi A. 2005. Pierwsza linia frontu. Postawy, doświadczenia zawodowe i kompetencje profesjonalistów pomagających ofiarom przemocy. [The first line of the front. Attitude, work experience and professional skills to assist victims of violence]. Niebieska Linia, 2, 26-29.

Rich, Ph. 2006. Attachment and sexual offending. Chichester: Wiley & Sons, Ltd.

Rocznik Demograficzny 2009 [The Demographic Yearbook of Poland 2009]. http://www.stat.gov.pl/gus/5840_3697_PLK_HTML.htm. (accessed January 30, 2010).

Rogulska, B. 2008. Społeczne przyzwolenie na bicie dzieci. Komunikat z badań, Centrum Badania Opinii Społecznej, www.cbos.pl. [Social approval of the beating of children. Communication of Research, Center for Public Opinion Research].

Ross, C.A., Duffy, CMM., Ellason, JW. 2002. Prevalence, reliability and validity of dissociative disorders in an inpatient setting. Journal of Trauma and Dissociation, 3, 7-17.

Ross, C.A. 2007. Borderline personality disorder and dissociation. Journal of Trauma and Dissociation, 8, 71-80.

Ross-Gower, J. Waller, G. Tyson, M. Elliott, P. 1998. Reported sexual abuse and subsequent psychopathology among women attending psychology clinics: The mediating role of dissociation. British Journal of Clinical Psychology, 37, 313-326.

Rothbaum, B.O., Foa, E.B., Riggs, D.S., Murdock, T., Walsh, W. 1992. A prospective examination of post-traumatic stress disorder in rape victims. Journal of Traumatic Stress, 5(3): 455-475.

Rothschild, B. 2000. The Body Remembers. The Psychophysiology of Truma and Trauma Treatment. London: W.W. Norton & Company.

Roy, M.A. 1977. Battered Women: A Psychosociological Study of Domestic Violence. New York: Van Nostrand Reinhold Company.

Rush, F. 1977. The Freudian cover-up. Chrysalis, 31-45.

Rusch, N., Weber, M., Il'yasov, KA. et al. 2007. Inferior frontal white matter microstructure and patterns of psychopathology in women with borderline personality disorder and comorbid attention-deficit hyperactivity disorder. Neuroimage, 35, 738-747.

Russ, M.J., Shearin, E.N., Clarkin, J.F., Harrison, K., Hull, J.W. 1993. Subtypes of self- injurious patients with borderline personality disorder. American Journal of Psychiatry, 150, 1869-1871.

Sachsse, U., Vogel, C., Leichsenring, F. 2006. Results of psychodynamically oriented trauma-focused inpatient treatment for women with complex posttraumatic stress disorder (PTSD) and borderline personality disorder. Bulletin of the Menninger Clinic, 70, 125-144.

Sakson-Obada, O. 2009. Pamięć ciała. Ja cielesne w relacji przywiązania i traumie. [Memory of the Body. Body ego in context of trauma and attachment.]. Warszawa: Wydawnictwo Difin.

Salter, A. 1988. Treating child sex offenders and victims. New York: Sage.

Salter-Ainsworth, M. 1993. Attachments and other affectional bonds across the life cycle. In M. Parkes, J. Stevenson – Hinde, P. Marris (Eds.), Across the Life Cycle (pp. 33 -52). New York: Routledge.

Sar, V., Akyuz, G., Kugu, N. et al. 2006. Axis I dissociative disorder comorbidity in borderline personality disorder and reports of childhood trauma. Journal of Clinical Psychiatry, 67:1583-1590.

Sar, V. Kundakci, T., Kiziltan, E. et al. 2003. The Axis-I dissociative disorder comorbidity of borderline personality disorder among psychiatric outpatients. Journal of Trauma and Dissociation, 4, 119-136.

Schauben, L. J. and P. A. Frazier. 1995. Vicarious trauma: The effects on female counselors of working with sexual violence survivors. Psychology of Women Quarterly, (19): 49-64.

Scheller-Gilkey, G., Moynes, K., Cooper, I., Kant, C., Miller, A.H. 2004. Early life stress and PTSD symptoms in patients with comorbid schizophrenia and substance abuse. Schizophrenia Research, 69 (2-3): 167-174.

Schier, K. 2009. Piękne brzydactwo. [Beautyiul ugliness]. Wydawnictwo: Scholar.

Schmahl, C. Bohus, M. Esposito, E. et al. 2006. Neural correlates of antinociception in borderline personality disorder. Archives of General Psychiatry, 63, 659-667.

Schmidt, N., Lerew, D.,Trakowski, J. 1997. Body vigilance in panic disorder: evaluating attention to body perturbations. Journal of Consulting and Clinical Psychology, 65: 214-220.

Seedat, S., Warwick, J., van Heerden, B. et al. 2004. Single photon emission computed tomography in posttraumatic stress disorder before and after treatment with a selective serotonin reuptake inhibitor. Journal of Affective Disorder, 80: 45-53.

Seligman, M. E. 1993. Optymizmu można się nauczyć. [Optimism can be learned.]. Poznań: Media i Rodzina.

Seligmann, M. E. 1974. Depression and learned helplessness. In Friedman M. M., Katz B. (Eds.), Psychology of Depression. Contemporary Theory and Research. Washington: Washington V. H.

Shearer, SL. 1994. Dissociative phenomena in women with borderline personality disorder. American Journal of Psychiatry, 151, 1324-1328.

Sierra, M., Berrios, GE. 1998. Depersonalization: neurobiological perspectives. Biological Psychiatry, 44, 898-908.

Simeon, D., Guralnik, O., Hazlett, E. et al. 2000. Feeling unreal: a PET study of depersonalization disorder. American Journal of Psychiatry, 157, 1782-1788.

Simeon, D., Knutelska, M., Smith, L., Baker, BR., Hollander, E. 2007. A preliminary study of cortisol and norepinephrine reactivity to psychosocial stress in borderline personality disorder with high and low dissociation. Psychiatry Research, 149, 177-184.

Simeon, D., Nelson, D., Elias, R., Greenberg, J., Hollander, E. 2003. Relationship of personality to dissociation and childhood trauma in borderline personality disorder. CNS Spectrums, 8, 755-757, 760-762.

Skowrońska, A. 2009. Doświadczenia małoletnich matek i ojców ich dzieci. Aspekty socjopedagogiczne. [The Experiences of Juvenile Mothers and Their Children's Fathers. Socjopedagogical Aspects.]. In R. Borowicz (Ed.), Współobecne dyskursy. [Co-present Discourses] (pp.413-436). Toruń: Wydawnictwo Uniwersytetu Mikołaja Kopernika.

Smith, C. 1996. The link between childhood maltreatment and teenage pregnancy. Social Work Research, 20: 131-142.

Spitzer, C., Barnow, S., Freyberger, H.J., Grabe, H.J. 2006. Recent developments in the theory of dissociation. World Psychiatry, 5(2): 82-86.

Stamm, B.H. 2002. Measuring compassion satisfaction as well as fatigue: Developmental history of the compassion satisfaction and fatigue test. In C.R. Figley (Ed.), Treating Compassion Fatigue (pp. 107-119). London: Taylor& Francis.

Stanik, J.M. 1980. Asocjalność nieletnich przestępców jako przedmiot psychologicznej diagnozy klinicznej. [Asocciality of juvenile offenders as a matter of psychological clinical diagnosis.]. Warszawa: Wydawnictwo Prawnicze.

Statystyka Sądowa i Penitencjarna Ministerstwa Sprawiedliwości. [Judicial Statistics of the Ministry of Justice and Penitentiary.]. 1998. Warszawa.

Staub, E., Volhardt, J. 2008. Altruism born of suffering: The roots of caring and helping after victimization and Rother trauma. American Journal of Orthopsychiatry, Vol. 78(3), 267-280.

Steinberg, M. 1994. Structured Clinical Interview for DSM-IV Dissociative Disorders, Revised (SCID-D-R). Washington, DC: American Psychiatric Press.

Stein, DJ., Hollander, E., DeCaria, CM. et al. 1996. M-chlorophenylpiperazine challenge in borderline personality disorder. Biological Psychiatry, 40, 508-513.

Stinson, D.A., Logel, C., Zanna, M.P., Holmes, J.G., Cameron, J.J., Wood, J.V., Spencer, S.J. 2008. The cost of lower self esteem: Testing a self- and social bonds model of heath. Journal of Personality and Social Psychology, Vol. 94(3), 412-423.

Stith, S., Rosen, K., Middleton, K., Busch, A., Lundeberg, K., Carlton, R. 2000. The Intergenerational Transmission of Spouse Abuse: A Meta-Analysis. Journal of Marriage and the Family, 62, 640-654.

Stover, C.S., Meadows, A.L., Kauffman, J. 2009. Interventions for intimate partner violence: Review and implications for evidence-based practice. Professional Psychology: Research and Practice, 40,3, 223-233.

Strelau, J., Zawadzki, B., Oniszczenko, W., Sobolewski, A., Pawłowski, P. 2004. Temperament i style radzenia sobie ze stresem jako moderatory zespołu stresu pourazowego w następstwie przeżytej katastrofy. [Temperament and coping with stress as moderators of PTSD as a result of lived disaster.]. In J. Strelau (Ed.., Osobowość a ekstremalny stress. [Personality and extreme stress.] (pp. 48-64). Gdańsk: Gdańskie Wydawnictwo Psychologiczne.

Suchańska, A. 1998. Przejawy i uwarunkowania psychologiczne pośredniej autodestruktywności. [Symptoms and psychological determinants of intermediate self-destructiveness.]. Poznań: Wydawnictwo Naukowe AUM.

Swartz, M., Blazer, D., George, L., Winfield, I. 1990. Estimating the prevalence of borderline personality disorder in the community. Journal of Personality Disorders, 4, 3, 257-272.

Szczepańska, J. 2008. Komu i jak pomagać? Pomoc społeczna w opinii Polaków. Komunikat z badań, Centrum Badania Opinii Społecznej. [To whom and how to help? Social assistance in the opinion of the Poles. Communication of Research, Center for Public Opinion Research.]. www.cbos.pl.

Tebartz, van Elst, I., Hesslinger, B., Thiel, T., et al. 2003. Frontolimbic brain abnormalities in patients with borderline personality disorder: a volumetric magnetic resonance imaging study. Biological Psychiatry, 54, 163-71.

Terr, L.C. 1988. What happens to early memories of trauma? Child and Adolescent Psychiatry, 27, 96-104.

—. 1991. Childhood trauma: An outline and overview. American Journal of Psychiatry, 148(1): 10-20.

Terr, L. 1994. Unchained memories: True stories of traumatic memories, lost and fund. New York: Basic Books.

Terzic, J., Mestrovic, J., Dogas, Z., Furlan, D. and Biocic, M. 2001. Children war casualties during the 1991-1995 wars in Croatia and Bosnia and Herzegovina. Croatian Medical Journal, 42(2): 156-160.

Tesch, R. 1990. Qalitative Research: Analysis Types and Software Tools. New York: The Falmer Press.

Thoma, H., Kachele, H. 1996. Podręcznik terapii psychoanalitycznej. [Handbook of psychoanalytic therapy.]. Warszawa: Pracownia Testów Psychologicznych PTP.

Tolin, D.F., Foa, E.B. 2006. Sex differences trauma and posttraumatic stress disorder: A quantitative review of 25 years research Psychological Trauma: Theory, Research, Practice, and Policy, Vol. S(1), 37-85.

Torinek, T., Katic, M., Kern, J. 2005. Morbidity of native, immigrant, and returned refugee populations in family medicine practice in Croatia after 1991-1995 war. Croatian Medical Journal, 46(6): 990-995.

Torgersen, S. Kringlen, E. Cramer, V. 2001. The prevalence of personality disorders in a community sample. Archives of General Psychiatry, 58, 590-596.

Torras de Bea, E. 1987. Body schema and identity. The International Journal Of Psycho-Analysis, 68: 175-84.

Van Den Bosch, LMC., Verheul, R., Langeland, W., Van Den Brink, W. 2003. Trauma, dissociation, and posttraumatic stress disorder in female borderline patients with and without substance abuse problems. Australian and New Zealand Journal of Psychiatry, 37, 549-555.

Van der Kolk, B. 1996a. The body keeps the score. Approaches to the psychobiology of post-traumatic stress disorder. In B.A. van der Kolk, A.C. McFarlane & L. Weisaeth (Eds.), Traumatic Stress. New York: Guilford.

—. 1996b. The complexity of adaptation to trauma: Self - regulation, stimulus discrimination, and characterologial development. In B.A. van der Kolk, A.C. Mc Farlane, and L. Weisaeth (Eds.), Traumatic stress: The effects of overwhelming experience on mind, body, and society (pp. 182-213). New York: Guilford Press.

—. 1999. The body keeps the score. In M.J. Horowitz (Ed.), Essential papers on Posttraumatic stress disorder. New York - London: New York University Press.

—. 2003. The neurobiology of childhood trauma and abuse. Child and Adolescent Psychiatric Clinics, 12: 293-317.

—. 2005. Developmental trauma disorder. Psychiatric Annals, 35, 401 - 408.

Van der Kolk B, Greenberg, M., Boyd, H., Krystal, J. 1985. Inescable shock, neurotransmitters, and addiction to trauma: toward a psychobiology of post traumatic stress. Biological Psychiatry, 20: 314-325.

Van Der Kolk, B., Roth, S., Pelcovitz, D., Sunday, S., Spinazolla, J. 2005. Disorders of extreme stress: The empirical foundation of a complex adaptation to trauma. Journal of Traumatic Stress, 18, 389 - 399.

Van der Kolk B., Saporta, J. 1993. Bological response to psychic trauma. International Handbook of Traumatic Stress Syndromes. New York and London: Plenum Press.

Van Hooff, M., Mc Farlane, A., Baur, J., Abraham, M., Barnes, D. 2009. The stressor Criterion-A1 and PTSD: a matter of opinion? Journal of Anxiety Disorder, 23, 1, 77-86.

Vukušić, H., Wilson, J.P., Gregurek, R., Komar, Z., Pavic, L., Gogic, B. 2003. Secondary victimization of war veterans with post-traumatic stres disorder: the Croatian experience. Psychiatria Danubina, 15(1-2): 13-25.

Walker, L. 1988. Battered women syndrome. In Hotaling G. T., Finkelhor D., Kirkpatrick J. T., Straus M. A. Family Abuse and its Consequences. Newbury Park: Sage Publication.

—. 2009. The Battered Woman Syndrome. New York: Springr Pub. Company.

Walker, R., Logan, T., Jordan, C. 2004. An integrative review of separation in the context of victimization. Consequences and implications for women. Trauma, Violence, & Abuse. A Review Journal, Vol. 5, 2, s. 143-194.

Wallen, R. 1963. Clinical Psychology. Warszawa: PWN.

Weather, F., Keane. T. 2007. Weathers' and Keane's, "the criterion A problem revisited: controversies and challenges in defining and measuring psychological trauma". Journal of Traumatic Stress, 20, 2, 107-121.

Weber, K., Rockstroh, B., Borgelt, J., Awiszus, B., Popov, T. 2008. Stress load during childhood affects psychopathology in psychiatric patients, BMC Psychiatry 63(8), http://www.biomedcentral.com.

Wenzel, M. 2005. Przemoc i konflikty w domu. Komunikat z badań. Warszawa. Centrum Badania Opinii Społecznej. [Violence and conflict at home. Communication from the study. Warsaw. Center for Public Opinion Research.]. www.cbos.pl.

—. 2009. Przemoc i konflikty w domu. Komunikat z badań. Warszawa. Centrum Badania Opinii Społecznej. [Violence and conflict at home. Communication from the study. Warsaw. Center for Public Opinion Research.]. www.cbos.pl.

Widera-Wysoczańska, A. 2000. Rozmowy o przemijaniu. Hermeneutyczne badanie psychologiczne. [Dialog about passing. Psychological hermeneutical research.]. Wroclaw: Uniwersytet Wrocławski Publ.

—. 2005. Zaburzone rodzicielstwo jako konsekwencja kazirodztwa doznanego w dzieciństwie. [Abnormal parenting as a rulet of incest experiened In childhood.]. Przegląd Psychologiczny [The Review of Psychology], 48, 3, 295-313.

—. 2006. Incest risk factors in the family: A Qualitative Study. Polish Journal of Applied Psychology, Vol. 4, N.1, 7 - 29.

—. 2006a. The influence of Chronic Trauma Experienced in Childhood on Womne's Heath (pp. 303-321). In A. Kuczynska, E. Dzikowska. (Eds.), Understanding Sex and Gender. Wrocław: Oficyna Wydwanicza ATUT.

—. 2007. Building healthy relationships: Integrated psychotherapy for persons after chronic childhood trauma. In Rudolf Gregurek (Eds.), Therapists' Affective Responses (197-236). Dubrownik.

—. 2010. Mechanizmy przemocy w rodzinie. Z pokolenia na pokolenie. [Mechanism of abuse in the family. From generation to generation]. Warszawa: Dyfin.

—. 2010a. Chronic, interpersonal trauma and integration psychotherapy

(in press).
—. 2010b. The risk factors of sexual abuse in the family (in preparing).
Widom, C.S. 1991. Avoidance of criminality in abused and neglected children. Psychiatry, 54, 162-174.
Widom, C.S., Ames, M.A. 1994. Criminal consequences of childhood sexual victimization. Child Abuse and Neglect, 18, 303-318.
Widom, C.S., Dutton, M.A., Czaja S.J., DuMont K.A. 2005. Development and Validation of a New Instrument to Assess Lifetime Trauma and Victimization History. Journal of Traumatic Stress, 18, 5, 519-531.
Widom, C. S., Kuhns, J. B. 1996. Childhood victimization and subsequent risk for promiscuity, prostitution, and teenage pregnancy: A prospective study. American Journal of Public Health, 86: 1607-1612.
Weiss, R. 1993. The attachment bond in childhood and adulthood. In M. Parkes, J. Stevenson – Hinde, P. Marris, (Eds.), Across the Life Cycle (pp. 66-77). New York: Routledge.
Więcławska, A. 2005. Nieletnie dziewczęta samotnie wychowujące dzieci a ich przygotowanie do radzenia sobie z ograniczeniami losu. [Underage Single Mothers and Their Ability to Manage the Fate Limitations.]. Toruń: Wydawnictwo Uniwersytetu Mikołaja Kopernika.
Wildgoose, A., Clarke, S., Waller, G., 2001. Treating personality fragmentation and dissociation in borderline personality disorder: a pilot study of the impact of cognitive analytic therapy. British Journal of Medical Psychology, 74, 47-55.
Wilkin, A. 1998. Wszystko powraca w snach. Długotrwałe konsekwencje psychologiczne klęski żywiołowej na przykładzie powodzi. [Everything comes back in dreams. Long-term psychological consequences of natural disasters on the example of flooding.]. Nowiny Psychologiczne, 1998: 3
Witwer, M. 1997. Early sexual activity, but not childhood sexual abuse, increases the odda of teenage pregnancy. Family Planning Perspectives, 29: 195-196.
Wojciszke, B.2000. Relacje interpersonalne. [Interpersonal relationships.]. In J. Strelau (Eds.), Psychologia. Podręcznik akademicki. [Psychology. Academic textbook.]. Tom III (pp. 147-204). Gdańsk: Gdańskie Wydawnictwo Psychologiczne.
Word Health Organization Global Consultation on Violence & Health. 1996. Violence: A public health priority (WHO/EHA/SPLPOA. 2). Geneva: Word Health Organization.
www.healthyteennetwork.org. (accessed August 23, 2009).
www.brpd.gov.pl/uploadfiles/publikacje/ekspertyza.pdf. (accessed September 1, 2009).

Wycisk, J. 2004. Okaleczanie ciała. [Body Self-Harm.]. Poznań: Bogucki Wydawnictwo Naukowe.

Yehuda, R., Davidson, J. 2002. Clinician's Manual on Posttraumatic Stress Disorder, London: Science Press.

Yehuda, R. 2003, Post-traumatic Stress Disorder. New England Journal of Medicine, 436(2): 108-14.

Zadumińska, B. 2006. Sytuacja ofiar zgwałcenia w postępowaniu przygotowawczym. Raport z monitoringu. Publikacja została przygotowana w ramach współpracy z Fundacją im. S. Batorego-Program Strażniczy. [The situation of rape victims in the trial proceedings. Monitoring Report. The publication was prepared in cooperation with the S. Batory Foundation.]. Kraków.

Zahm, D.S. 2000. An integrative neuroanatomical perspective on some subcortical substrates of adaptive responding with emphasis on the nucleus accumbens. Neuroscience & Biobehavioral Review, 24(1): 85-105.

Zakrzewska, E. 2001. Budowanie systemu przeciwdziałania przemocy domowej w Olsztynie - na przykładzie działań Miejskiego Zespołu Profilaktyki i Terapii Uzależnień. Rola Ośrodków Pomocy Społecznej we wspieraniu osób uzależnionych i ofiar przemocy. X Ogólnopolska Konferencja Stowarzyszenia Samorządowych Ośrodków Pomocy Społecznej. [Building a system of domestic violence in Olsztyn - a case study of the Municipal Team for Prevention and Therapy of Addiction. In: The Role of Social Welfare Centres in helping drug addicts and victims of violence. X National Conference of the Association of Municipal Social Welfare Centrem.]. Olsztyn.

Zanarini, M.C., Frankenburg, F.R., Jager-Hyman, S., Reich, D.B., Fitzmaurice, G. 2008. The course of dissociation for patients with borderline personality disorder and axis II comparison subjects: a 10-year follow-up. Acta Psychiatrica Scandinavica, 118, 291-296.

Zanarini, M.C., Ruser, T.F., Frankenburg, F.R., Hennen, J.H., 2000. Risk factors associated with the dissociative experiences of borderline patients. Journal of Nervous and Mental Disease, 188, 26-30.

Zimbardo, P.G., Ruch, F.L. 1997. Psychologia i życie. [Psychology and life.]. Warszawa: Wydawnictwo Naukowe PWN.

Zubieta, J.K., Chinitz, J.A., Lombardi, U., Fig, L.M., Cameron, O.G. and Liberzon, I. 1999. Medial frontal cortex involvement in PTSD symptoms: a SPECT study. Journal of Psychiatric Research, 33: 259-264.

Zweig-Frank, H. Paris, J. Guzder, J. 1994a. Dissociation in female patients with borderline and non-borderline personality disorders. Journal of Personality Disorders, 8, 203-209.

Zweig-Frank, H. Paris, J. Guzder, J. 1994b. Dissociation in male patients with borderline and non-borderline personality disorders. Journal of Personality Disorder.

CONTRIBUTORS

Maria Beisert, lawyer, psychologist and clinical sexologist - Professor, PhD, researcher at the Institute of Psychology University named after A. Mickiewicz in Poznań. Head of the Laboratory of Clinical and Social Sexology, and Head of the Psychological Assistance Postgraduate Studies in the Field of Sexology at the Institute of Psychology at the University of Poznań. Her most important books include *The sex of your child*, *Divorce*, *The process of coping with crisis*, *Incest*, *Parents as perpetrators*, and *Sexuality in the life cycle*.

Lidia Cierpiałkowska, PhD, is a Professor at A. Mickiewicz University in Poznań. Her main field of specialization is clinical psychology and psychotherapy. Current research interest focuses on the verification of assumptions of object relation theory related to levels of personality organizations (psychotic, borderline and neurotic) and to personality disorders in alcoholics. She is the author of *Psychopathology*, *Alcoholism: Self-help Groups and Professional Therapy*; *Psychology of Addictions: Alcoholism.*

Paul F. Dell, PhD is former Professor of Psychiatry and Behavioral Sciences, Eastern Virginia Medical School; recipient of the International Society for the Study of Trauma and Dissociation's Morton Prince Award for Scientific Achievement (2004) and the Pierre Janet Writing Award (2006). Co-editor of Dell and O'Neil (2009), *Dissociation and the Dissociative Disorders: DSM-V and Beyond.*

Dorota Dyjakon, Ph.D., is assistant professor in the Unit of Sciences on the Family at the University of Lower Silesia, a psychotherapist, author of the book *Violence, therapy, gratification* (2010) and of several articles among which are *The autobiographical interview as a way of getting to know changes in identity* (2005), *Influence of the psychotherapy on changes in relations of family alcoholics who perpetrate domestic violence"* (2006), *Overcoming trauma: a narration in the process of psychotherapy* (2007).

Rudolf Gregurek, MD, PhD, Prof., is head of tye Clinic for Psychological Medicine, Clinical Hospital Centre Zagreb, head of the Desk for Psychiatry and Psychological Medicine, University of Zagreb Medical School.

Marilyn Korzekwa, Dr, received her MD degree from the University of Toronto in 1982 and completed psychiatry residency at McMaster University in Hamilton in 1986, where she is an assistant professor. She is acting director of the Dialectical Behavior Therapy (DBT) Day Hospital at St. Joseph's Hospital. She has published numerous papers about Borderline Personality Disorder (BPD) and is a member of the International Study for the Study of Trauma and Dissociation.

Alicja Kuczyńska, clinical and social psychologist - professor, PhD, head of the Department of Clinical and Health Psychology at the Institute of Psychology, Wrocław University. She is editor of the Polish Journal of Applied Psychology. Her main field of interest is concerned with human bonding in social and personal relationships, from an evolutional and social theories point of view (e.g. sex and gender as well as other nonverbal aspects). For about the last ten years she has been focusing her interest on borderline personality disorders.

Beata Pastwa-Wojciechowska, PhD, is a Professor of Forensic and Clinical Psychology at the Institute of Psychology at University of Gdańsk, where she is Dean of the Faculty of Social Sciences. She also works at Court in Gdańsk as a psychological expert. She wrote chapters or articles in English: *Comorbidity of ADHD and psychopathy symptoms in men violating legal standards. Acta Neuropsychologica*, 6(4), 325-336, (2005); *Perception of one's own and another person's behavior related to morality in groups of noncriminals and psychopaths*, in A. Czeredrecka, T. Jaśkiewicz-Obydzińska, R. Roesch, J. Wójcikiewicz (eds), *Forensic Psychology and Law. Facing the Challenges of a Changing World* (41-65), Kraków, Institute of Forensic Research Publishers, (2008) *The significance and role of sex among psychopathic perpetrators of the crime of incest* (pp. 228-248), in: A. Cybicka, S.F. Safdar, A. Kwiatkowska (eds.), (2010).

Irena Pospiszyl, Professor in Social Pathology, Head of Department of Social Pathology at Academy of Social Rehabilitation in Warsaw, 115 Marszałkowska Street, Poland. Publications/ books;(2000) *"Przemoc w rodzinie" (Intimate violence)*, Warsaw, ed. WSiP; (1997) "Przemoc w instytucjach opiekuńczo-wychowawczych" (*Abuse in Educational Institutions* - edr.), Warsaw, ed. WSPS ,IBE; (2009) - *"Patologie społeczne" (Social Pathology)* Warsaw, ed; (2003) - *Ofiary chroniczne (Chronic victims*), Warsaw ed. APS.

Olga Sakson-Obada, PhD, is a psychologist, a lecturer in the Institute of Psychology at Adam Mickiewicz University, Poznań. She specializes in trauma and body ego. She is an author of book *Body ego in trauma and attachement.*

Alicja Strzelecka-Lemiech, PhD., psychologist and psychotherapist, having completed training in process-oriented therapy, Gestalt therapy, movement therapy, and work with the body. She runs a private practice (counseling, crisis intervention, and psychotherapy) and also develops workshop and vocational training programs (including those involving domestic violence).

Agnieszka Widera-Wysoczańska, PhD, is a Clinical Psychologist, Adjunct Professor in the Clinical Department, Intitute of Psychology, Wrocław University, Poland and Co-Developer of the Mental Health Center for Persons from Dysfunctional Families. She specializes in interpersonal, chronic and complex childhood trauma in dysfunctional families and in the risk factors of sexual abuse in the families. She is a Psychotherapist of the European Psychotherapy Association, Trauma Specialist, Supervisor in diagnosis and therapy for people after trauma, and Consultatnt in Child Clinical Psychology. She was a member of the National Agency Against Family Violence (2007 - 2009). She has authored books entitled *Dialog About Dying: Hermeneutical Approaches* (2000) and *Mechanism of Abuse in the Family. From Generation to Generation* (2010), and has published numerous articles on related topics.

Jowita Wycisk, PhD, is a psychologist, a graduate of cultural studies, a lecturer in Institute of Psychology at Adam Mickiewicz University (Poznań). Her scientific interests are psychology of gender, personal and cultural factors determining self-injury behaviours, and psychological aspects of teenage motherhood.